Diseases of the Inner Ear

Masoud Motasaddi Zarandy
John Rutka

Diseases of the Inner Ear

A Clinical, Radiologic and Pathologic Atlas

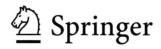 Springer

Masoud Motasaddi Zarandy, MD
Professor
Tehran University of Medical Sciences
Amiralam Hospital
Cochlear Implant Dept.
Saadi Ave.
Tehran
Iran
motesadi@sina.tums.ac.ir

John Rutka, MD, FRCSC
Professor
University of Toronto
Dept. Otolaryngology-Head and Neck
Centre for Advanced Hearing
200 Elizabeth St.
Toronto ON M5G 2C4
Canada
john.rutka@uhn.on.ca

ISBN: 978-3-642-05057-2   e-ISBN: 978-3-642-05058-9

DOI: 10.1007/978-3-642-05058-9

Springer Heidelberg Dordrecht London New York

Library of Congress Control Number: 2010920823

Cover design: eStudio Calamar, Figueres/Berlin

Printed on acid-free paper

Springer is part of Springer Science+Business Media (www.springer.com)

Preface

It is by your own eyes and your ears and your own mind and (I may add) your own heart that you must observe and love

Sir William Osler

It has been just over 20 years that Hawke and Jahn's seminal book entitled *Diseases of the Ear: Clinical and Pathologic Aspects* was published. The book was unique from other textbooks in otology at the time and concentrated its message according to two well-known proverbs in English literature namely "*A picture is worth a thousand words*" and "*Seeing is believing.*"

Dr. Masoud Motasaddi Zarandy has taken these twin concepts, and in the process, has produced a very beautiful and a visually pleasing book. The pictures and accompanying text allows the reader not only to see how different pathologies affect the inner ear but also to appreciate the clinical consequences that arise from our decision-making processes. Far from dry, the inner ear and skull base comes to life when we see the dynamics of how disease involves this complex and integral part of the body.

For the uninitiated, this book takes us on a tour of the field that has evolved over the past decade into the formal discipline of neurotology/skull base medicine and surgery. It has quite rightly become a specialized branch of otolaryngology/neurosurgery where interdisciplinary collaboration has become the rule rather than the exception. Advances in imaging (including intraoperative stereotaxis), technology (i.e., implantation for profound sensorineural hearing loss), and molecular biology have all played a role in the further management of disorders in this region and will continue to do so in future.

With regard to its content, the book is divided into a number of chapters that cover the clinical conditions that commonly involve the inner ear and skull base. To mention a few of the chapters in the book provides case in point. For example, the histopathology of temporal bone malignancy is a rarely ever appreciated *antemortem*, yet it continues to provide us with a wealth of information concerning how tumors spread in the skull base. Our understanding of congenital deafness and its association with various developmental inner ear anomalies have significant practical consequences regarding the success or failure of cochlear implantation surgery. The success of physical therapy maneuvers for the treatment of benign positional paroxysmal vertigo might realistically depend on whether the patient has cupulolithiasis or canalolithiasis as the pathologic cause. All the above considerations are detailed in the accompanying text.

As Dr. Motasaddi's principal mentor during his fellowship at the University of Toronto, I have had an extremely gratifying experience to have been a small part of his overall growth as a physician and surgeon. His book contains the pure essence of clinical research, which compels us forward in the hopes that we may better care for our patients in the treatment of their disorders. As in any endeavor, there were a number of individuals who helped in one way or another. In this regard, the authors specifically thank Professor Blake Papsin and Dr. Susan Blaser for providing us with the necessary imaging that helped improve our understanding of inner ear anomalies. We would also be remiss if we did not acknowledge the pioneering work of Professor Michael Hawke (the world's foremost chronicler of otologic pathology), whose beautiful otoscopic pictures grace this book. Finally, we thank all those who were involved in the Ear Pathology Research Laboratory at the University of Toronto over the years. While the lab somewhat sadly is no longer in existence, its archival collection contains an unparalleled source of unique medical information to this day. And who ever thought old bones couldnot tell new tales!

Finally, the quote at the beginning of this preface from Sir William Osler, father of modern medicine, continues to ring true for all medical practitioners. May this book in conjunction from what you hear and learn from your patients continue to guide you in your mission to heal!

Toronto, Canada   Prof. John Rutka

Contents

Core Messages

> Temporal bone malignancies are a heterogeneous collection of tumors and rarely diagnosed when asymptomatic.

> Mechanisms of spread include direct extension, hematogenous dissemination, perineural spread and/or CSF dissemination.

> Hematogenous dissemination frequently involves the petrous apex.

> Differential diagnosis for metastatic spread in acute or progressive cochleovestibular/facial nerve dysfunction should be considered when a background history of remote malignancy exists.

Metastatic carcinoma of the temporal bone is uncommon and is documented in the literature mostly by single-case reports and several small series.

The pathology is rarely recognized initially, because it can be either asymptomatic or overshadowed by other metastases in the disease course. Involvement of the temporal bone usually occurs late in the disease process.

History and physical examination as well as a high index of suspicion are paramount in the diagnosis of metastatic carcinoma of the temporal bone [5, 6].

Symptoms of metastatic carcinoma to the temporal bone in a patient with remote malignancy can include otorrhea, pain, hearing loss, tinnitus, vertigo, disequilibrium, and facial nerve paralysis. The onset of symptoms may be acute or progressive, appearing early or late in the disease course. Temporal bone metastasis may be occult and asymptomatic or occasionally the first clinical manifestation of the primary malignancy. Although uncommon, the

clinician must include metastases of a carcinoma to the temporal bone in the differential diagnosis of any acute or progressive cochleovestibular or facial nerve dysfunction, especially in patients with a history of carcinoma [6].

Sites for primary tumors are most commonly the breast, lung, kidney, stomach, bronchus, and prostate. They can also be primarily hematogenous (i.e., leukemia) [1, 6] (Figs. 1.1–1.7).

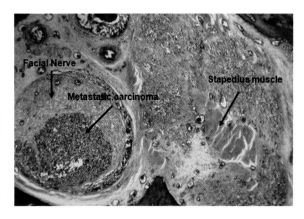

Fig. 1.1 Breast cancer with metastasis to the facial nerve

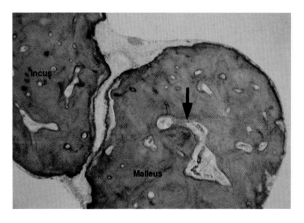

Fig. 1.2 Breast cancer with metastasis to the malleus

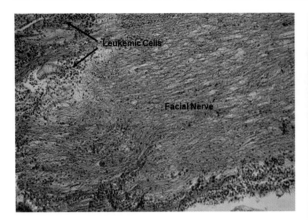

Fig. 1.3 Acute lymphocytic leukemia (*ALL*) demonstrating facial nerve involvement

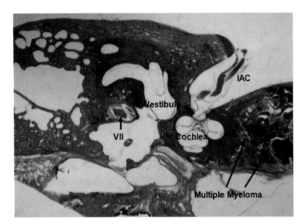

Fig. 1.4 Multiple myeloma and temporal bone involvement in the petrous apex

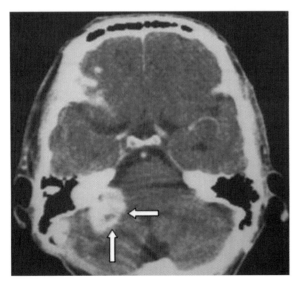

Fig. 1.5 Renal cell carcinoma with metastasis to the CP angle which mimicked an acoustic neuroma. See *arrows*

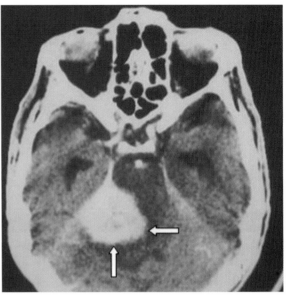

Fig. 1.6 Renal cell carcinoma with metastasis to the CP (same patient as in Fig. 1.5). See *arrows*

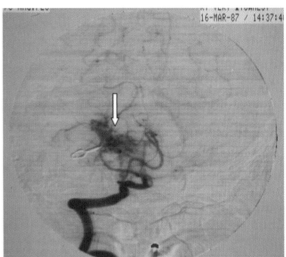

Fig. 1.7 Selective carotid angiogram demonstrating tumor blush from metastatic renal cell carcinoma. Angiographic findings can occasionally mimic a glomus jugulare tumor. See *arrow*

For all hematogenously spread metastatic tumors, the most common site of involvement within the temporal bone is the petrous apex followed by the tegmen (middle cranial fossa dural plate), mastoid bone, and internal auditory canal (IAC) [1].

Temporal bone metastases from noncontiguous, distant primary lesions are thought to occur via the following mechanisms:

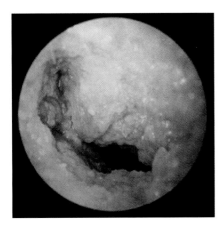

Fig. 1.8 Squamous cell carcinoma of the ear canal

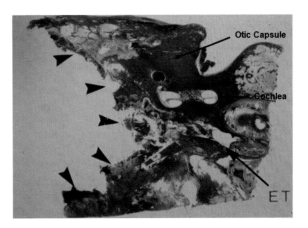

Fig. 1.11 Direct temporal bone invasion by squamous cell carcinoma. See *arrows*. The otic capsule remains relatively well preserved despite the extensive erosion. *ET* eustachian tube

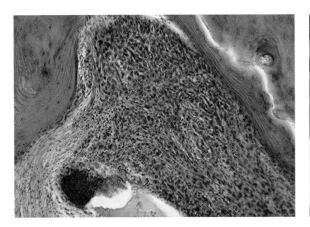

Fig. 1.9 Squamous cell carcinoma infiltrating the petrous apex

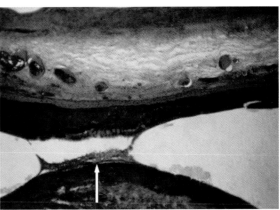

Fig. 1.12 Squamous cell carcinoma involving the eustachian tube. See *arrow*

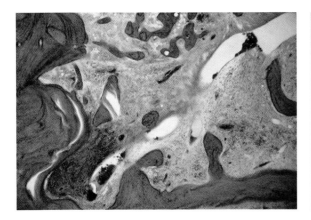

Fig. 1.10 Infiltrative squamous cell carcinoma to the petrous apex. The carcinoma has created islands of bone

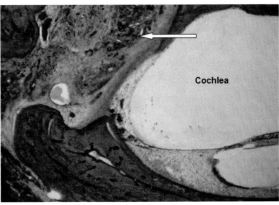

Fig. 1.13 Squamous cell carcinoma involving the cochlea. See *arrow*

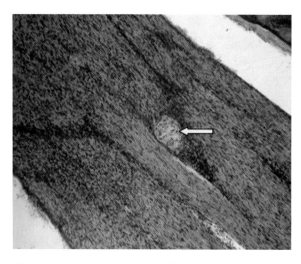

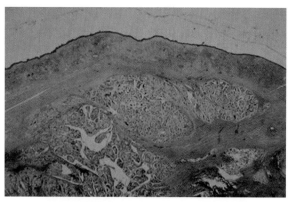

Fig. 1.16 Temporal bone involvement by adenoid cystic carcinoma. Tumor often metastases by direct extension from the parotid gland or via perineural spread

Fig. 1.14 Metastatic squamous cell carcinoma involving the facial nerve. See *arrow*

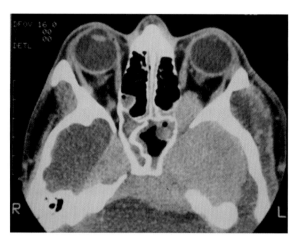

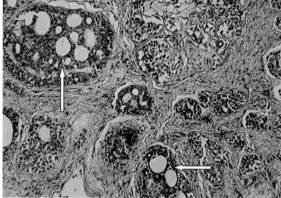

Fig. 1.17 Adenoid cystic carcinoma demonstrating the so-called "Swiss Cheese" appearance. See *arrows*

Fig. 1.15 CT scan demonstrating invasive nasopharyngeal squamous cell carcinoma involving skull base with extension into the temporal bone

1. Hematogenous spread of carcinoma with seeding of the marrow spaces of the petrous bone.
2. Cerebrospinal fluid dissemination through the subarachnoid space and into the IAC resulting in temporal bone invasion [5, 6].

Once in the temporal bone, there are two distinct modes of tumor spread: (a) vascular-osseous (petrous apex, mastoid, middle ear, and external canal); and (b) perineural (nerves in IAC branches, and labyrinthine end-organs) or both [4] (Figs. 1.8–1.33).

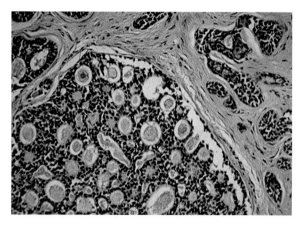

Fig. 1.18 Adenoid cystic carcinoma demonstrating perineural involvement

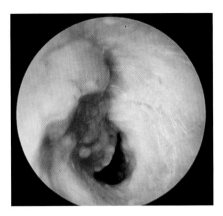

Fig. 1.19 Adenoid cystic carcinoma directly extending into the external auditory canal arising from the parotid gland

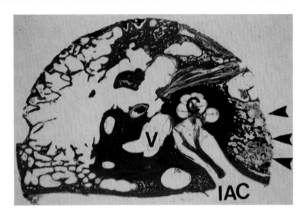

Fig. 1.21 Hematogenous spread of carcinoma to the petrous apex. See *arrows* (*V* vestibule; *C* cochlea; *IAC* internal auditory canal)

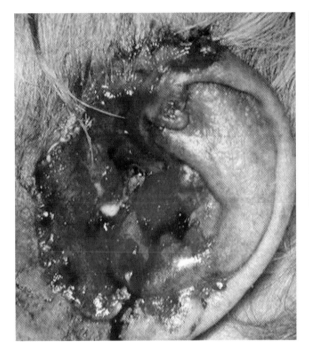

Fig. 1.20 Basal cell carcinoma with direct extension into the temporal bone

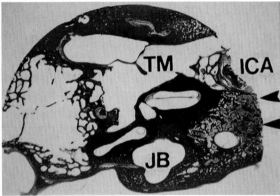

Fig. 1.22 Hematogenous spread of carcinoma to the petrous apex (see *arrows*). The otic capsule appears relatively well preserved. Same patient as in Fig. 1.15 (*JB* jugular bulb; *TM* tympanic membrane; *ICA* internal carotid artery)

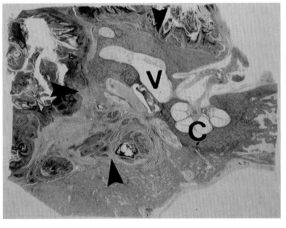

Fig. 1.23 Widespread involvement of the temporal bone by carcinoma (see *arrows*). Note the relative preservation again of the otic capsule (*V* vestibule; *C* cochlea)

The diagnosis of a metastasis to the temporal bone is typically overshadowed by other complaints a patient with metastatic carcimona may have. Discharge from the ear is often mistaken for a chronic otitis media/externa when in fact the carcinoma is causative. When the dura becomes involved, the pain becomes severe and unrelenting. Development of a cochleovestibular loss and facial palsy are ominous findings. A high-resolution computed tomography (CT) scan of

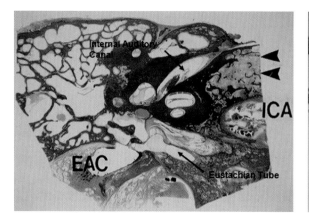

Fig. 1.24 Primary involvement of the porus acousticus, internal carotid artery and eustachian tube by metastatic carcinoma. See *arrows* (*ECA* external auditory canal; *ICA* internal carotid artery)

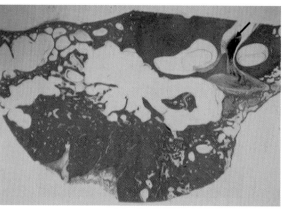

Fig. 1.27 Metastatic malignant melanoma in the internal auditory canal involving the facial nerve

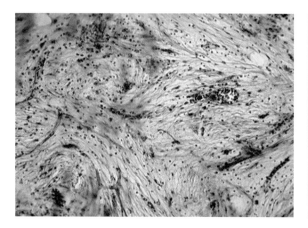

Fig. 1.25 Leukemic infiltration

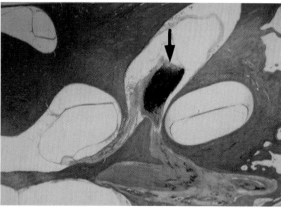

Fig. 1.28 Malignant melanoma in the internal auditory canal involving the facial nerve. Note the involvement of the geniculate ganglion as well. See *arrow*

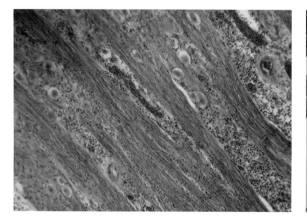

Fig. 1.26 Leukemic infiltration to the superior vestibular nerve

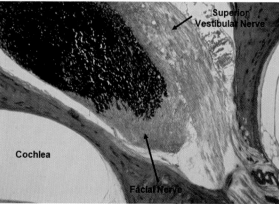

Fig. 1.29 Malignant melanoma within the internal auditory canal

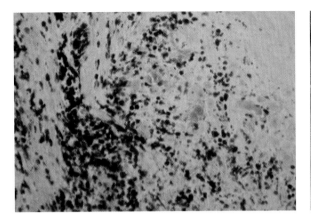

Fig. 1.30 Melanotic cells

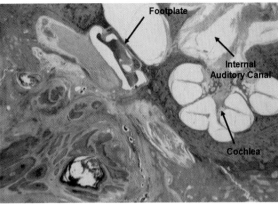

Fig. 1.32 Verucous carcinoma and the temporal bone. Tumor has eroded the ossicular chain. Stapes footplate still preserved

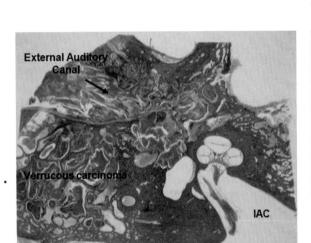

Fig. 1.31 Verrucous carcinoma of the temporal bone. Described as a locally invasive yet pathologically benign lesion, it behaves clinically like a malignancy. Bone invasion is typically through the routes of least resistance such as the mastoid air cells. The otic capsule again seems relatively well preserved. Note the complete involvement IAC internal auditory canal of the mastoid air cell system and the external auditory canal

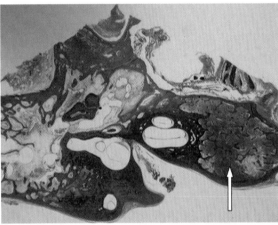

Fig. 1.33 Histiocytosis of the petrous apex. See *arrow*

References

1. Belal A Jr (1985) Metastatic tumours of the temporal bone. A histopathological report. J Laryngol Otol 99(9):839–846
2. Berlinger NT, Koutroupas S, Adams G, Maisel R (1980) Patterns of involvement of the temporal bone in metastatic and systemic malignancy. Laryngoscope 90(4):619–627
3. Feinmesser R, Libson Y, Uziely B, Gay I (1986) Metastatic carcinoma to the temporal bone. Am J Otol 7(2):119–120
4. Jahn AF, Farkashidy J, Berman JM (1979) Metastatic tumors in the temporal bone – a pathophysiologic study. J Otolaryngol 8(1):85–95
5. Nelson EG, Hinojosa R (1991) Histopathology of metastatic temporal bone tumors. Arch Otolaryngol Head Neck Surg 117(2):189–193
6. Streitmann MJ, Sismanis A (1996) Metastatic carcinoma of the temporal bone. Am J Otol 17(5):780–783

the head and temporal bones is mandatory as part of the complete investigation. While CT is excellent in the delineation of bony lesions, involvement of the IAC and posterior fossa is probably best seen with a magnetic resonance imaging scan [3, 6]. The prognosis is especially poor in epithelial derived metastatic carcinomas (i.e., squamous cell carcinoma).

Cholesteatoma and Its Complications

2

Core Messages

> Major properties of cholesteatoma include bone erosion and secondary infection.

> Both congenital and acquired cholesteatoma can cause intratemporal and intracranial complications.

> Recidivistic rates (residual and recurrent disease) are higher in childhood cholesteatoma.

> Mastoid surgery is required to provide a safe, dry and when possible better hearing ear.

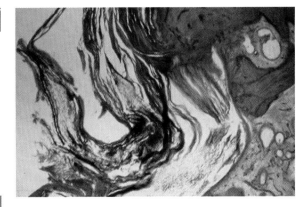

Fig. 2.1 Cholesteatoma (note its destructive effect on bone)

Cholesteatoma is a term whose initial use can be credited to Muller in 1838. The first case, however, of a cholesteatoma-like mass was reported by Du Verneey in 1683, who described a mass between the cerebellum and the cerebrum. In essence, the term cholesteatoma represents the presence of the stratified squamous epithelium within the middle ear space that clinically has two significant properties, namely secondary infection and bone erosion (Fig. 2.1).

It is accepted that cholesteatoma may be either congenital or acquired [8]. To date, several pathogenic mechanisms have been proposed to explain the pathogenesis of cholesteatoma. Proposed theories of congenital cholesteatoma include: (a) the presence of an ectopic epidermis rest, (b) in-growth of meatal epidermis, (c) metaplasia following infection/inflamation, and somewhat interestingly, (d) reflux of amniotic fluid containing squamous epithelium in utero into the middle ear (Fig. 2.2).

The actual incidence of congenital cholesteatoma is difficult to determine. Nevertheless, greater awareness among physicians has occurred with the introduction

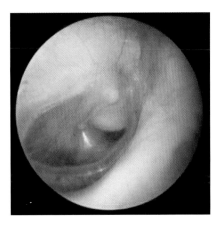

Fig. 2.2 Congenital cholesteatoma. Typically presents as a whitish mass (Michael's body) in epitympanum behind an intact tympanic membrane

of the high resolution CT and MRI. Perhaps as a result, its incidence seems to be increasing [5, 10].

Unlike primary acquired cholesteatoma, congenital cholesteatoma typically does not present with a prior

M. M. Zarandy and J. Rutka, *Diseases of the Inner Ear*
DOI: 10.1007/978-3-642-05058-9_2, © Springer-Verlag Berlin Heidelberg 2010

history of otorrhea, tympanic membrane perforation, or previous surgery. While there is hearing loss (usually conductive initially), the tympanic membrane is typically normal. With a close inspection, however, a pearly white mass (so-called Michael's body) medial to the ear drum is often noted [5, 7].

At the other end of the disease spectrum, the clinical picture of a child with otorrhea, hearing loss (conductive type), a tympanic membrane perforation in an atypical location together with a mastoid filled with cholesteatoma also may represent the end point in the natural history of congenital cholesteatoma. Distinguishing between congenital and acquired cholesteatoma is, however, not always that obvious [6].

Proposed theories for the pathogenesis of acquired cholesteatoma, include: (a) invaginations of the tympanic membrane from chronic Eustachian tube dysfunction resulting in retraction pockets (primary acquired cholesteatoma), (b) basal cell proliferation, (c) epithelial in-growth into the middle ear through a perforation (the immigration theory), (d) or inadvertent implantation (following myringotomy or tympanoplasty surgery), and (e) squamous metaplasia of the middle ear epithelium secondary to chronic infection/inflammation/persistent use of ototopical agents [8] (Figs. 2.3–2.5).

Congenital cholesteatoma of the temporal bone may be divided into four anatomic areas for consideration: (1) middle ear, (2) petrous apex, (3) perigeniculate area, and (4) primary cerebellopontine angle and combinations thereof [1].

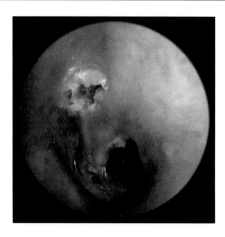

Fig. 2.4 Primary acquired cholesteatoma. Cholesteatoma is thought to arise from retraction pockets with the failure of epithelial migration leading to keratin accumulation and the development of a gradually expanding sac. A history of a chronic, painless, and malodorous discharging ear is not unusual

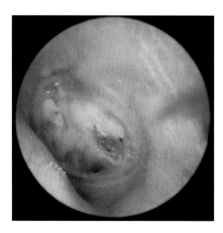

Fig. 2.5 Acquired cholesteatoma. Implantation of the squamous epithelium lead to the development of cholesteatoma after tympanoplasty

The most common sites of presentation on physical examination are behind the anterior-superior and posterior–superior quadrants of the tympanic membrane.

While conductive hearing loss tends to be the most common presenting symptom, perigeniculate and petrous apex cholesteatomas are not infrequently present with an insidious or rapidly progressive facial nerve paralysis [5].

Bone erosion and secondary infection from cholesteatoma can lead to both intratemporal (facial paralysis, infective cochleolabyrinthitis, etc.) and intracranial complications (meningitis, brain abscess, sigmoid sinus

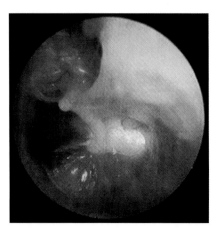

Fig. 2.3 Primary acquired cholesteatoma. Retraction pockets in the pars flaccida from chronic Eustachian tube dysfunction lead to the development of a keratin containing sac within the middle ear

thrombophlebitis, etc.) in both congenital and acquired forms of the disease.

Occasionally, a patient with congenital cholesteatoma may present with complications of the disease. Complications of congenital cholesteatoma that arise from bone erosion not infrequently involve the facial nerve at the level of the geniculate ganglion and its labyrithine segment. Despite significant erosion into the otic capsule, partial hearing and vestibular function are not infrequently maintained [13].

Bilateral congenital cholesteatoma is a rare condition but has been reported [7] (Figs. 2.6–2.10).

In general, intracranial complications are more likely to arise in primary acquired cholesteatoma as a result of secondary infection. Erosion into the otic capsule of the lateral semicircular canal is frequently identified in primary acquired cholesteatoma where disease spread usually follows an orderly pattern through a route of least resistance via the aditus ad antrum, antrum, and into the mastoid bone proper (Figs. 2.11–2.25).

Cholesteatoma is still considered a surgical disease requiring either the complete removal of its squamous lined matrix or its exteriorization for continued aural toilet and ventilation. To this end, different tympanomastoidectomy procedures are available.

Surgery for cholesteatoma is generally divided into combined approach tympanomastoidectomy (canal wall up) or modified radical and radical (canal

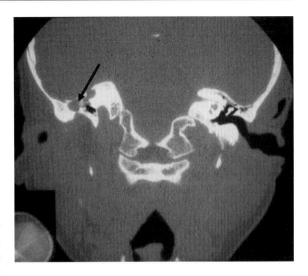

Fig. 2.7 Congenital cholesteatoma. Note the smooth bony erosions in the anterior epitymanum typical for cholesteatoma. See *arrow*

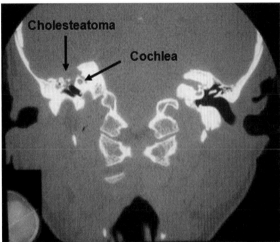

Fig. 2.8 Congenital cholesteatoma demonstrating erosion into the cochlea. Patient presented with an acute facial nerve paralysis and a longstanding sensorineural hearing loss. Vestibular function was partially intact

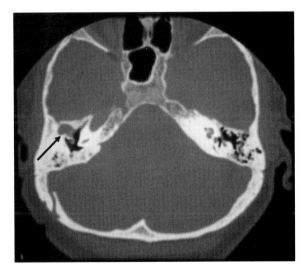

Fig. 2.6 Congenital cholesteatoma (*arrow*). Typically presents as a mass in the epitympanum behind an intact tympanic membrane

wall down) mastoidectomy procedures. The first and foremost goal of surgery is to provide a safe, dry and when possible, a better hearing ear. Reconstruction of the ossicular chain (ossiculoplasty) often depends on the remaining anatomy of the middle ear and Eustachian tube function. Hearing results in congenital cholesteatoma frequently depend on its location and the significant involvement of the ossicular chain.

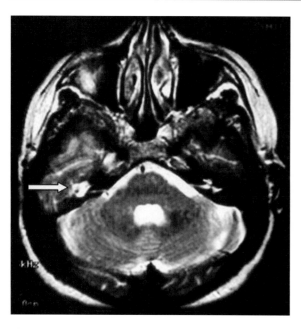

Fig. 2.9 MRI T2-weighted image demonstrating congenital cholesteatoma (see *arrow*). Relative magnitude of hydrogen atoms in keratin causes it to assume a bright fluid-like signal similar to cerebrospinal fluid

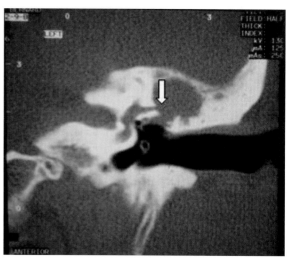

Fig. 2.11 Primary acquired cholesteatoma causing erosion with fistula into the lateral semicircular canal (see *arrow*). Axial CT scan

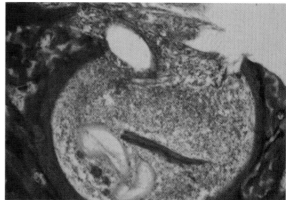

Fig. 2.12 Acute bacterial labyrinthitis from cholesteatoma involving the lateral semicircular canal

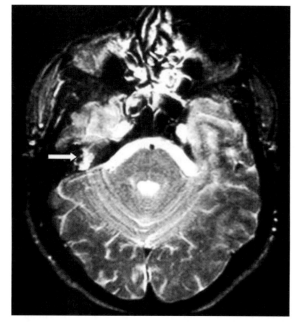

Fig. 2.10 MRI image of intralabyrinthine cholesteatoma (*arrow*)

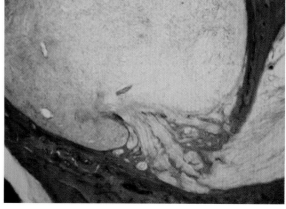

Fig. 2.13 Acute bacterial labyrinthitis involving the superior semicircular canal from cholesteatoma

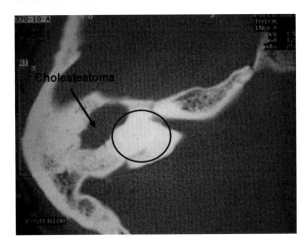

Fig. 2.14 Axial CT scan. Labyrinthitis ossificans of the cochlea and labyrinth following acute labyrinthitis caused by cholesteatoma. Note the absence of inner ear structures. See *black circle*

When restricted to the epitympanum, good results in hearing following surgery are often possible especially if the cholesteatoma is diagnosed and treated early [3, 11, 12].

From the world literature, it would appear that the best treatment results in childhood cholesteatoma are obtained in the early clinical stage. Open procedures (i.e., atticotomy, modified radical mastoidectomy, etc.) seem to have the best long-term results. However, canal wall up procedures have been recommended as the first-line surgical option in children. Nevertheless, the recidivistic (residual and recurrent disease) rate tends to be higher. Each case therefore needs to be evaluated separately and the appropriate technique should be tailored to the individual patient's needs and surgical expectations [4, 5].

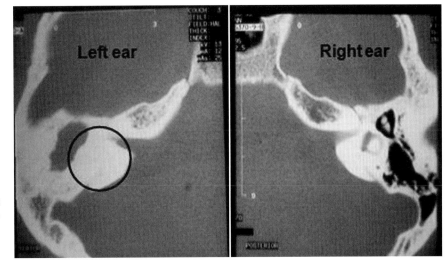

Fig. 2.15 Labyrinthis ossificans (see *circle*) secondary to cholesteatoma in the left ear (same patient as in Fig. 2.14). Note the normal lateral *SCC* and ossicles in right ear

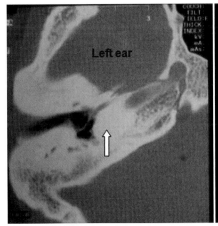
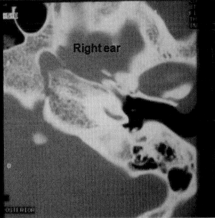

Fig. 2.16 Labyrinthitis ossificans from cholesteatoma (same patient as in Figs. 2.14 and 2.15). Note the absence of cochlea in the left ear compared to the right side

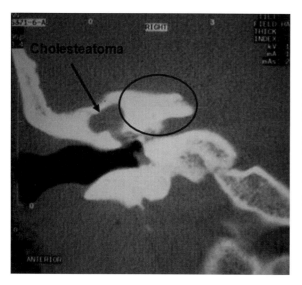

Fig. 2.17 Coronal CT scan demonstrating labyrinthitis ossificans of semicircular canals (see *circle*) (same patient as in Figs. 2.14 and 2.15)

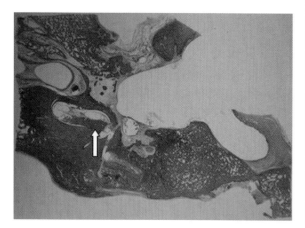

Fig. 2.18 Labyrinthitis ossificans from cholesteatoma. The ossification process (osteoneogenesis) usually starts in the basal turn of the cochlea closest to the round window membrane. See *arrow*. Note that a previous mastoidectomy had been performed

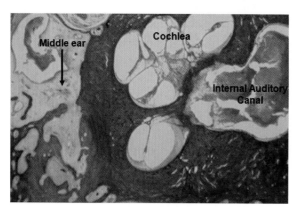

Fig. 2.19 Meningitis secondary to cholesteatoma

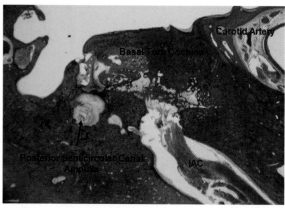

Fig. 2.20 Labyrinthitis ossificans demonstrating osteoneogenesis postmeningitis. The patient survived the meningitis but developed a complete cochleovestibular loss

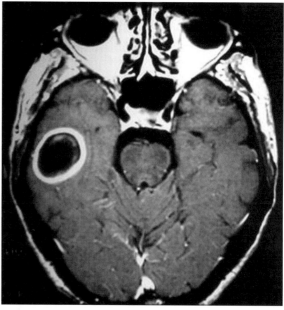

Fig. 2.21 Intracranial complication of cholesteatoma. Temporal lobe brain abscess. secondary to cholesteatoma

Petrous apex cholesterol granulomas share many similar clinical features with cholesteatomas in the petrous apex. However, their pathogenesis appears very different. A cholesterol granuloma specifically represents a foreign body granulomatous response to cholesterol crystals in the submucosal tissues of air cells in the temporal bone. While cholesterol granulomas are frequently found in patients with chronic otitis media, it is thought that petrous apex cholesterol

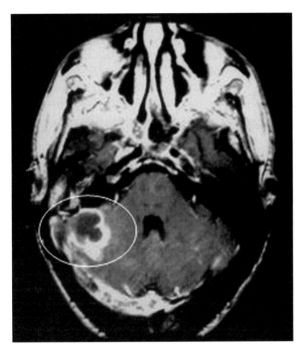

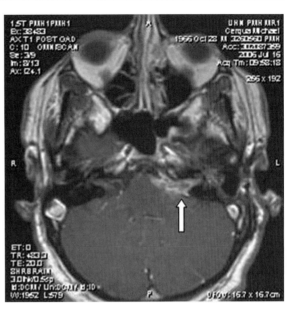

Fig. 2.24 Intracranial complication. Abscess in the internal auditory canal secondary to cholesteatoma (see *arrow*)

Fig. 2.22 Intracranial complications of cholesteatoma. Cerebellar abscess and sigmoid sinus thrombophlebitis (see *circle*) as complications of cholesteatoma

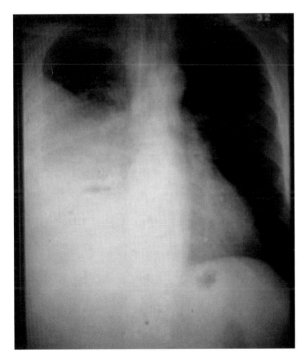

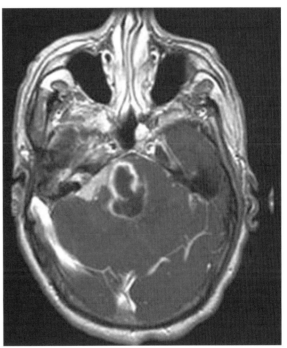

Fig. 2.25 Intracranial complication. Pontine abscess secondary to cholesteatoma

granulomas arise when a normally pneumatized air cell becomes isolated from it air supply.

Progressive growth of a petrous apex cholesterol granuloma may result in a petrous apex syndrome with diplopia from the abducens nerve involvement and the

Fig. 2.23 Lung abscess secondary to infected thromboemboli from sigmoid sinus thrombophlebitis (same patient as in Fig. 2.21). Le Meriere's disease is used to describe this phenomenon

trigeminal and facial nerve palsies. The onset of the sensorineural hearing loss and vertigo implies erosion into the inner ear. Treatment requires extensive surgical drainage following the pneumatized perilabyrinthine air cell tracts surrounding the otic capsule when inner ear function is present. However, recurrences are not infrequent and multiple surgeries are often required [2, 9] (Figs. 2.26–2.31).

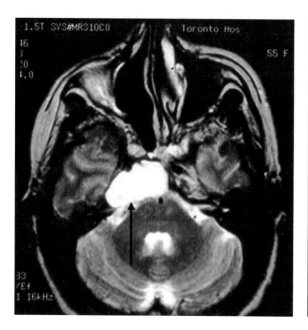

Fig. 2.26 MRI scan demonstrating clival epidermoid (*arrow*). Example of a congenital rest of epithelial cells remote from the middle ear and mastoid

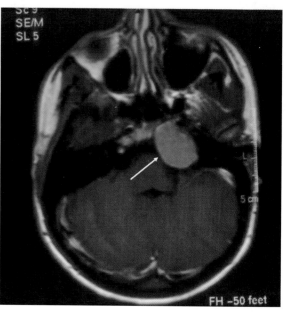

Fig. 2.28 MRI scan demonstrating a large left petrous apex cholesterol granuloma in a patient presenting with diplopia from an abducens nerve palsy. See *arrow*

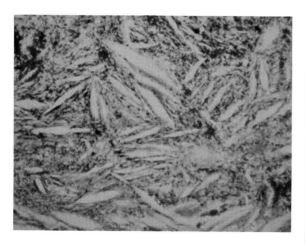

Fig. 2.27 Cholesterol granulomas are characterized by numerous empty, ovoid, slit-like spaces that are surrounded by foreign body giant cells and fibrous tissue

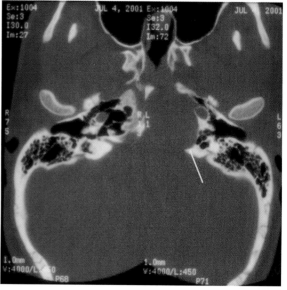

Fig. 2.29 CT demonstrating smooth expansile mass in the petrous apex. Same patient as in Fig. 2.28. See *yellow arrow*

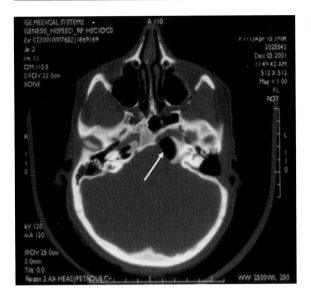

Fig. 2.30 Postoperative axial CT scan demonstrating aeration of the petrous apex following mastoid and infralabyrinthine drainage. See *yellow arrow*

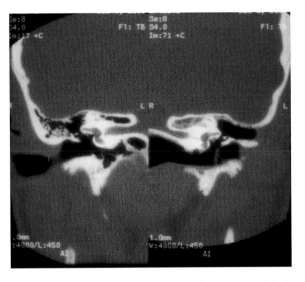

Fig. 2.31 Postoperative coronal CT scan demonstrating infralabyrinthine approach for drainage

References

1. Cummings CW (1991) Otolaryngology, head and neck surgery. In: Chronic otitis media, mastoiditis, and petrositis, 3rd edn. Mosby, Philadelphia
2. Edamatsu H, Aoki F, Misu T, Yamaguti H, Tokumaru A, Watanabe K, Fukazawa T (2002) Navigation-aided surgery for congenital cholesteatoma at the petrous apex. Nippon Jibiinkoka Gakkai Kaiho 105(12):1212–1215
3. Faramarzi A, Motasaddi-Zarandy M, Khorsandi MT (2008) Intraoperative finding in revision chronic otitis media surgery. Arch Iran Med 11(2):196–199
4. Karmody CS, Byahatti SV, Blevins N, Valtonen H, Northrop C (1998) The origin of congenital cholesteatoma. Am J Otol 19(3):292–297
5. Kazahaya K, Potsic WP (2004) Congenital cholesteatoma. Curr Opin Otolaryngol Head Neck Surg 12(5):398–403
6. Koltai PJ, Nelson M, Castellon RJ, Garabedian EN, Triglia JM, Roman S, Roger G (2002) The natural history of congenital cholesteatoma. Arch Otolaryngol Head Neck Surg 128(7):804–809
7. Kuczkowski J, Babinski D, Stodulski D (2004) Congenital and acquired cholesteatoma middle ear in children [Polish]. Otolaryngol Pol 58(5):957–964
8. Lesinskas E, Kasinskas R, Vainutiene V (2002) Middle ear cholesteatoma: present-day concepts of etiology and pathogenesis [Lithuanian]. Medicina (Kaunas) 38(11):1066–1071; quiz 1141
9. Nelson M, Roger G, Koltai PJ, Garabedian EN, Triglia JM, Roman S, Castellon RJ, Hammel JP (2002) Congenital cholesteatoma: classification, management, and outcome. Arch Otolaryngol Head Neck Surg 128(7):810–814
10. Nishizaki K, Yamamoto S, Fukazawa M, Yuen K, Ohmichi T, Masuda Y (1996) Bilateral congenital cholesteatoma. Int J Pediat Otorhinolaryngol 34(3):259–264
11. Okano T, Iwanaga M, Yonamine Y, Minoyama M, Kakinoki Y, Tahara C, Tanabe M (2004) Clinical study of congenital cholesteatoma of the middle ear [Japanese]. Nippon Jibiinkoka Gakkai Kaiho 107(11):998–1003
12. Sudhoff H, Liang J, Dazert S, Borkowski G, Michaels L (1999) Epidermoid formation in the pathogenesis of congenital cholesteatoma – a current review [German]. Laryngorhinootologie 78(2):63–67
13. Zarandy MM, Rajati M, Khorsandi MT (2007) Recurrent meningitis due to spontaneous cerebrospinal fluid otorrhea in adults. Int J Pediatr Otorhinolaryngol 3:113–116

Anomalies of the Inner Ear

3

Core Messages

> Imaging abnormalities are seen in 20% of patients with a congenital sensorineural hearing loss.

> Malformations can involve the cochlea, vestibule, semicircular canals or internal auditory canal alone or in combination.

> Incomplete partition II (IP-II) is synonymous with a Mondini's deformity.

> The severity of the malformation generally depends on the timing of the gestational development arrest.

Hearing loss from malformations of the auditory system may arise from morphologic abnormalities of the external canal, the middle ear, or the inner ear. Various combinations are possible. Overall, approximately 20% of patients with congenital sensorineural hearing loss have radiographic abnormalities of the inner ear.

The audiometric assessment together with the high-resolution computerized tomography (CT) and magnetic resonance imaging (MRI) of the temporal bone now makes it possible to obtain precise diagnostic evaluation of the inner ear malformations.

Developmental anomalies of the inner ear have been better characterized since the high-resolution CT scan has been used for the evaluation of cochlear implant candidates. These anomalies have been classified by several authors based on the radiologic anatomy and the presumed embryogenesis of the inner ear [7, 10, 13].

In general, the severity of any inner ear anomaly is believed to depend on the timing of the developmental arrest [7] (Figs. 3.1–3.10).

Anomalies of the inner ear can be divided as follows:

1. Cochlear malformations
2. Vestibular malformations
3. Semicircular canal malformations
4. Internal auditory canal (IAC) malformations

3.1 Cochlear Malformations

3.1.1 Michel Deformity

In 1863, Michel reported the first case of bilateral complete bony and membranous aplasia of the inner ear. Today, the complete absence of all cochlear and vestibular structures represents the hallmark of this eponymous malformation.

According to the classic theories of inner ear embryogenesis, the otic placode differentiates into the structures which will become the inner ear during the third week of gestation. Complete inner ear aplasia is thought to arise when development arrests before this time.

Michel aplasia clearly differs from Michel dysplasia. In the latter, the developmental arrest that results in dysplasia occurs later in gestation.

In general, labyrinthine aplasia is a very rare cause of congenital hearing loss. It is estimated that Michel's aplasia constitutes only 1% of cochlear bony malformations. When present, it may be unilateral or bilateral. While rare, it may run in families [2]. The incidence of complete inner ear aplasia, however, may

Fig. 3.1 Embryology of the inner ear. The inner ear begins its development from an invagination of the ectoderm with transformation of the otic placode into the otic vesicle

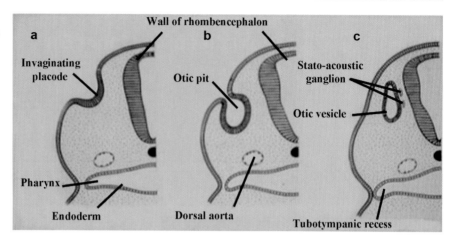

Fig. 3.2 Normal developing anatomy of the inner and middle ear. The inner ear embryologically develops before the middle ear

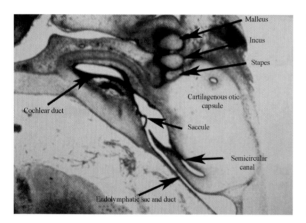

Fig. 3.4 Normal developmental anatomy later in gestation. Note the developing external auditory canal and the middle ear (eustachian tube, ossicular chain, and facial nerve) as mesenchyme remodels. The tubotympanic pouch is derived from the endoderm

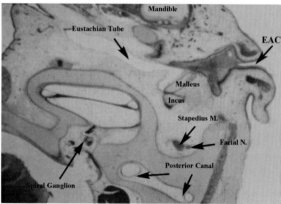

Fig. 3.3 Normal developmental anatomy. Inner ear development precedes the development of the middle ear

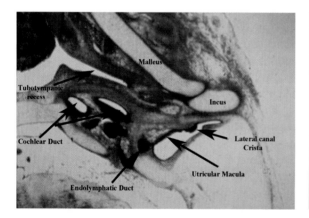

Fig. 3.5 Normal developmental anatomy. With further gestation the development of the inner ear is complete. Middle-ear structures are starting to approach maturity

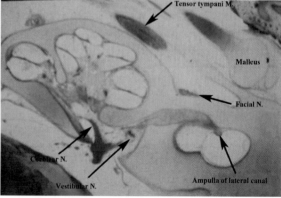

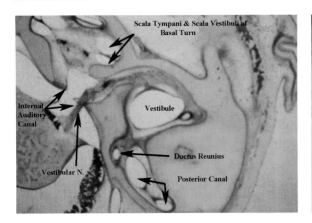

Fig. 3.6 Normal developmental anatomy of the basal turn of the cochlea and the vestibular apparatus

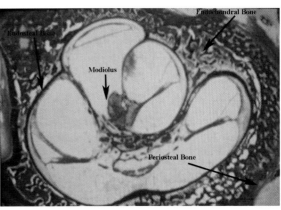

Fig. 3.8 Normal developmental anatomy of the cochlea and the otic capsule

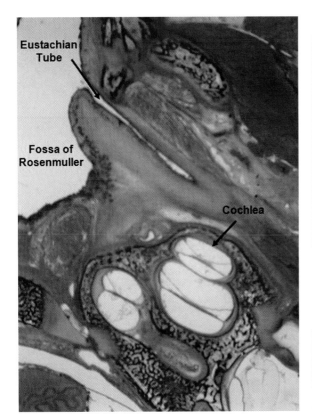

Fig. 3.7 Normal developmental anatomy of the cochlea in the later stages of development. Otic capsule becoming ossified as membranous labyrinth matures. Eustachian tube has completed its development

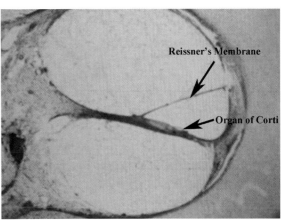

Fig. 3.9 Normal developmental anatomy of the membranous cochlea

be somewhat overestimated from radiographic reports as it may be confused with ossification of labyrinth (labyrinthitis ossificans) which is usually an acquired abnormality (Fig. 3.11).

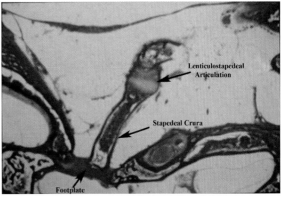

Fig. 3.10 Normal developmental anatomy of the stapes, stapes footplate, and facial nerve

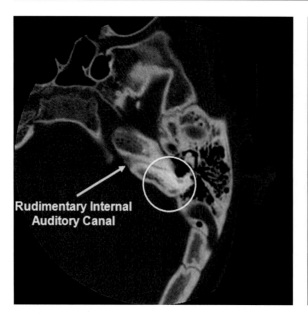

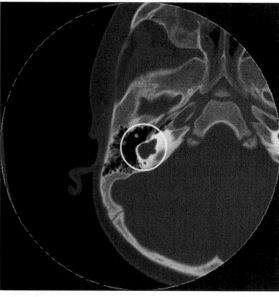

Fig. 3.11 Michel cochlear aplasia and external auditory meatus atresia. Note the absence of the inner ear (see *circle*) and the presence of a rudimentary internal auditory canal

Fig. 3.12 Axial CT scan of the common (cochlea – vestibular) cavity deformity. See *circle*

3.1.2 Cochlear Aplasia

In this anomaly, the cochlea is completely absent. There may be a normal, dilated, or hypoplastic vestibule and semicircular canals. Cochlear aplasia is diagnosed when a focus of dense otic bone is identified to involve the anterior part of the IAC. In the absence of the cochlea, the course of the labyrinthine segment of the facial canal is typically more anterior to its usual location. It is important to differentiate this malformation from secondary cochlear ossification (osteoneogenesis). In cochlear osteoneogenesis, while there is complete ossification of the cochlea, the basal turn of the cochlea produces some degree of bulging into the middle ear (the promontory), and the bony area in front of the IAC is of normal dimensions. However, in the aplastic cochlea, no bulging of the promontory is present.

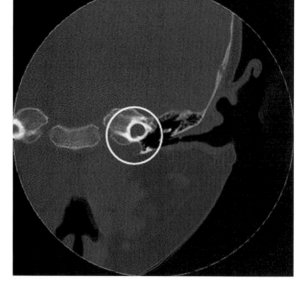

Fig. 3.13 A coronal CT image showing a common cavity anomaly. See *circle*

3.1.3 Common Cavity Deformity

In this variant, an undifferentiated cystic cavity or otocyst representing the cochlea and vestibule is identified (Figs. 3.12–3.14).

3.1.4 Cochlear Hypoplasia

In this variant, the malformation appears more differentiated. The cochlea and vestibule are separate from

Fig. 3.14 Postoperative cochlear implant CT images showing implant electrodes in a common cavity

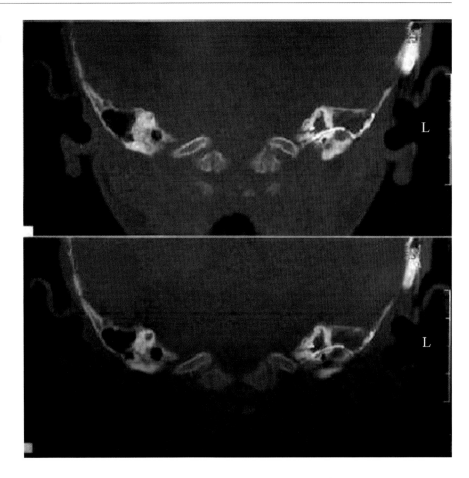

3.1.5 Incomplete Partition Type I (IP-I)

In the IP I, the cochlea lacks the entire modiolus and cribiform area has a cystic appearance. A large cystic vestibule is usually identified (Fig. 3.18).

3.1.6 Incomplete Partition Type II (IP-II) (Mondini Deformity)

Mondini's description of an inner ear abnormality bearing his name dates to 1791. Today it is generally accepted that a Mondini deformity (malformation) consists of one-and-half coils of the cochlea (instead of the normal two-and-half coils), a flattened cochlea with the development of the basal coil only, cystic dilatation of the common apical chamber with absence of the interscalar septum between the middle and apical coil, and a hypoplastic modiolus. A developmental arrest at the sixth week of embryonic life is believed to be responsible for the defect. Rarely is the defect bilateral. The vestibular structures may be abnormal as well. A spectrum of osseous and membranous abnormalities within the inner ear appear typical.

Occasionally some sensory epithelium can be found which provides hope that some hearing might be present. Inner ear malformations are not infrequently associated with other phenotypic syndromes. A diagnosis for a Mondini deformity should be suspected especially in children with deafness and/or recurrent bouts of meningitis [4, 11, 14] (Figs. 3.19–3.31).

each other but their dimensions are smaller than normal. The hypoplastic cochlea resembles a small bud off the IAC (Figs. 3.15–3.17).

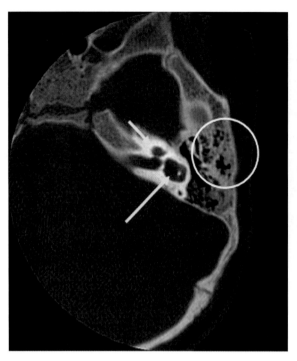

Fig. 3.15 Axial CT scan. Hypoplastic right cochlea (*small arrow*), external auditory meatus atresia (see *circle*) and a very small island of lateral semicircular canal (*large arrow*)

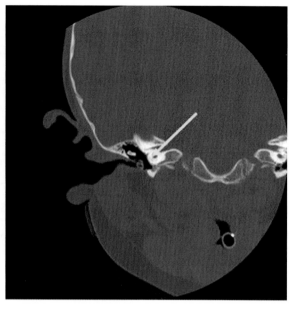

Fig. 3.17 Coronal CT scan. Hypoplastic cochlea (coronal section). See *yellow arrow*

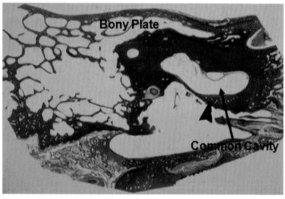

Fig. 3.18 Incomplete partition type 1 (IP-1). Common cavity is noted with the cystic attempt to develop inner ear. Bony plate prevents cochleovestibular nerve bundle from reaching the common cavity

3.2 Malformations of the Vestibule

Malformations of the vestibule are typically found in the Michel deformity and the common cavity defect. The spectrum of abnormalities may include an absent vestibule, a hypoplastic vestibule, or a dilated vestibule.

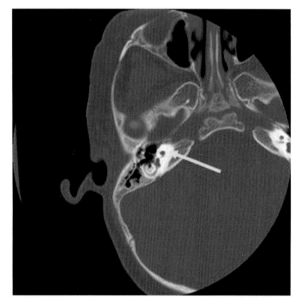

Fig. 3.16 Axial CT scan. Hypoplastic left cochlea (see *arrow*)

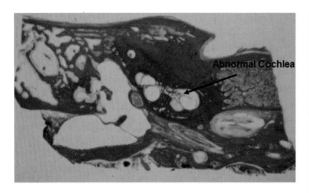

Fig. 3.19 Mondini deformity. Note the abnormal cochlea with one-and-half turns and failure of the neural structures in the internal auditory canal to reach the abnormal cochlea

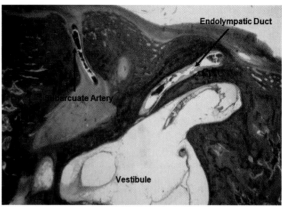

Fig. 3.22 Mondini deformity demonstrating an enlarged endolymphatic duct entering into the vestibule

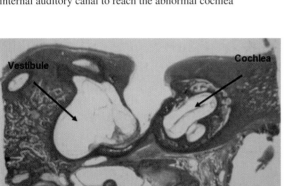

Fig. 3.20 Mondini deformity. (abnormal vestibule and cochlea)

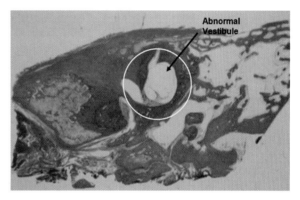

Fig. 3.23 Mondini deformity (abnormal vestibule). See *circle*

3.4 Internal Auditory Canal Malformations

IAC malformations are described as absent, narrow, or enlarged (Figs. 3.35–3.37).

Malformations of the IAC are not infrequently accompanied by other radiological abnormalities affecting the entire inner ear [3]. When a malformation of the IAC occurs, it is often associated with major deformities of the labyrinth specifically at the fundus. An abnormal communication of the CSF with the tympanic cavity can result in frequent bouts of meningitis (Fig. 3.38).

Congenital stenosis of the IAC is a rare cause of sensorineural hearing loss in children. Chief presenting symptoms besides hearing loss can include facial nerve palsy, dizziness, and tinnitus [1].

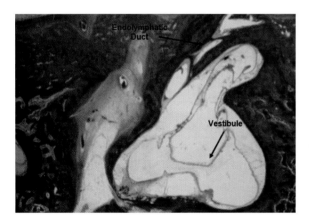

Fig. 3.21 Mondini deformity (abnormal vestibule)

3.3 Semicircular Canal Malformations

Semicircular canal malformations are described as absent, hypoplastic, or enlarged (Figs. 3.32–3.34).

Fig. 3.24 Mondini deformity. Widened vestibule left side (*yellow arrow*). One-and-half turns of cochlea right side (*white arrow*)

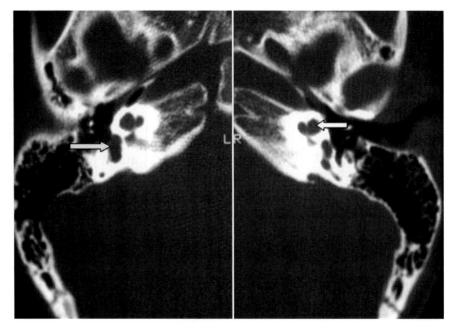

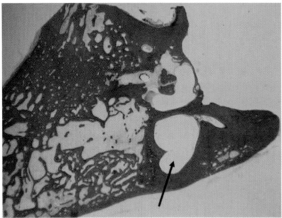

Fig. 3.25 Common cavity deformity. See Figs. 3.12 and 3.13

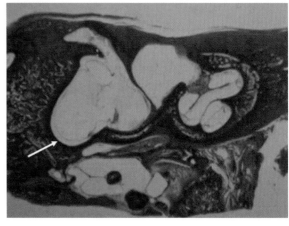

Fig. 3.27 Mondini deformity with enlarged vestibule (*arrow*)

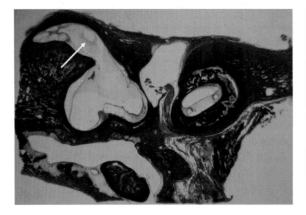

Fig. 3.26 Mondini deformity with posterior semicircular canal (*arrow*)

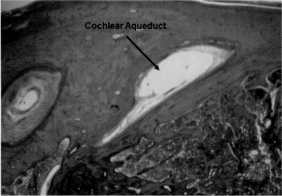

Fig. 3.28 Mondini deformity with normal cochlear aqueduct

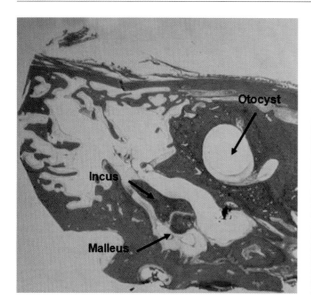

Fig. 3.29 Common cavity deformity. Circular appearance of otocyst with rudimentary neuroepithelium. See Figs. 3.12, 3.13 and 3.25

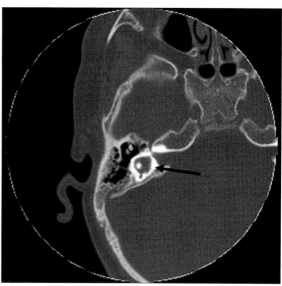

Fig. 3.32 Dilated vestibule. Small lateral semicircular canal, small bone island, and enlarged vestibule (*arrow*)

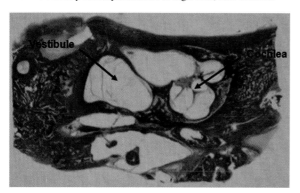

Fig. 3.30 Mondini deformity. Widened vestibule, two turns of the cochlea (left ear) only

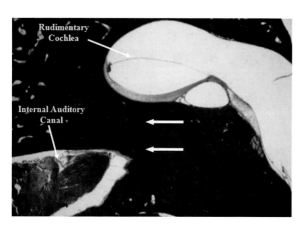

Fig. 3.31 Rudimentary attempt at cochlear formation. Single-turn cochlea noted. Abnormal internal auditory canal. Bony plate prevents innervation of the inner ear. See *arrows*

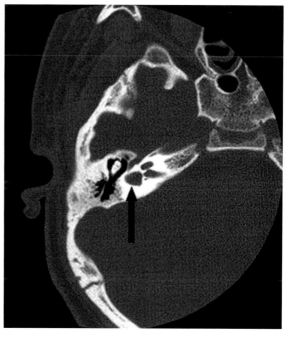

Fig. 3.33 Right inner ear abnormality in a Down's syndrome patient. Note the absence of the lateral semicircular canal. See *arrow*

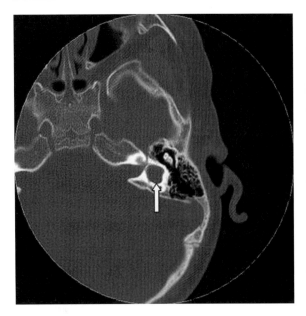

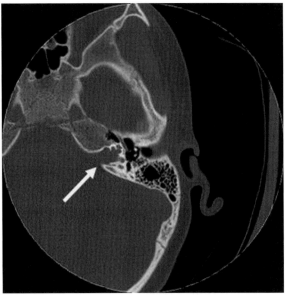

Fig. 3.34 Inner ear abnormality (absent lateral semicircular canal) in a Down's syndrome patient (same patient)

Fig. 3.36 Abnormal internal auditory canal (*arrow*) and vestibular hypoplasia. Note the direct communication with cochlea

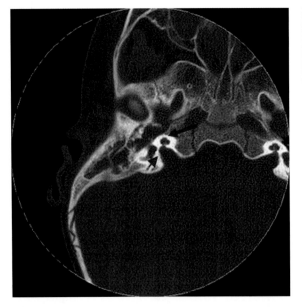

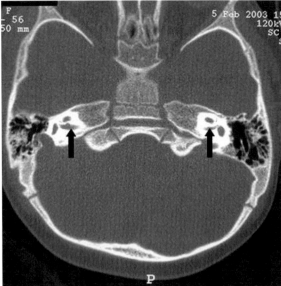

Fig. 3.35 Large internal auditory canal diameter (*arrowhead*) and hypoplastic cochlea in a patient with branchio-oto-renal syndrome (*arrow*)

Fig. 3.37 Hypoplastic internal auditory meati. See *arrows*

In the CHARGE syndrome, a number of inner ear abnormalities can be identified. CHARGE is an acronym referring to children with a specific pattern of birth defects. In short, the acronym is as follows: "C" for coloboma, "H" for heart defects, "A" for atresia choanae, "R" for retardation of growth and development, "G" for genitourinary problems, and "E" for ear abnormalities. The ear anomalies can affect the external ear (which may present with an unusually large of small and/or unusual shape of the external ear), middle

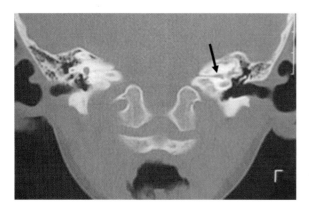

Fig. 3.38 Narrow internal auditory canal (Riley–Day syndrome) (*arrow*) (coronal CT scan)

An enlarged vestibular aqueduct syndrome is a relatively common congenital inner ear anomaly responsible for some unusual vestibular and audiological symptoms. Most cases show bilateral early onset and subsequent progressive hearing loss. The gross appearance on the CT scan of the inner ear is generally normal. However, when precise measurements of the inner ear components are performed, they often reveal abnormal dimensions (especially the endolymphatic duct) which may be responsible for the accompanying auditory and vestibular dysfunction [7, 9, 12] (Figs. 3.40, 3.41).

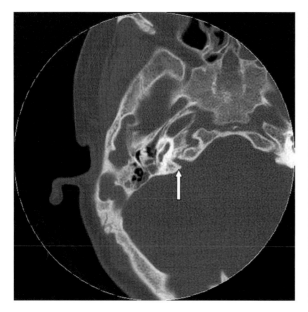

Fig. 3.39 CHARGE syndrome patient demonstrating a hypoplastic internal auditory canal. See *arrow*

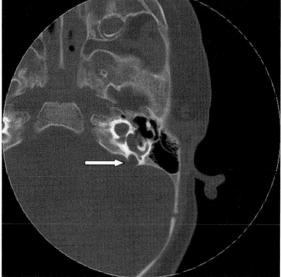

Fig. 3.40 Cochlear deformity associated with large vestibular aqueduct. See *arrow*

ear (bone malformations or chronic glue-ear), and/or the internal ear (especially high frequency hearing loss). A mixed hearing loss (conductive and sensorineural) is most frequently seen, i.e., from middle-ear problems and cochlear abnormalities (Fig. 3.39).

3.5 Vestibular and Cochlear Aqueduct Findings

Vestibular and cochlear aqueduct abnormalities are typically described as enlarged [6, 8, 10].

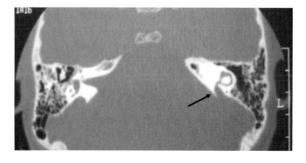

Fig. 3.41 Enlarged vestibular aqueduct (axial CT scan) (*arrow*)

3.6 Associated with Syndromes

3.6.1 Klippel–Feil Syndrome

The Klippel–Feil syndrome (KFS) has a reported incidence of 1/42,000 individuals. It may be transmitted by sporadic, autosomal dominant or autosomal recessive mechanisms.

The syndrome originally described by Klippel and Feil in 1912 consists of a congenital spinal malformation characterized by the failure in segmentation of 2 or more cervical vertebrae. Although the anomaly is defined by its skeletal component, KFS can also be associated with the developmental defects in many other organ systems including the inner ear, spinal cord, heart, and genitourinary tract. Abnormalities in the usual course and relationships of the facial nerve to other middle ear and mastoid structures often occurs [5] (Figs. 3.42–3.44).

The following pages in this chapter demonstrate other temporal bone abnormalities (Figs. 3.45–3.54).

Figures 3.11–3.17, 3.24, 3.32–3.47 are shown in this atlas courtesy of Dr. Blake Papsin.

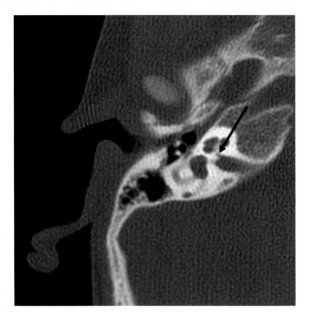

Fig. 3.43 CT image of a hypoplastic eighth cranial nerve (*arrow*)

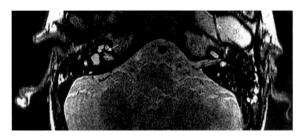

Fig. 3.44 Hypoplastic eighth cranial nerve. See *arrow*

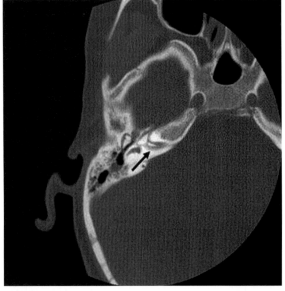

Fig. 3.42 Duplicate seventh cranial nerve from the internal auditory canal (*arrow*)

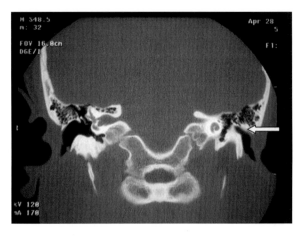

Fig. 3.45 Abnormal left external auditory canal. See *arrow*

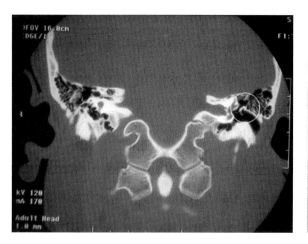

Fig. 3.46 Abnormal incus and malleus of the left ear. Coronal CT. See *circle*

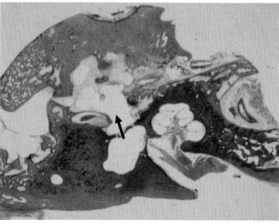

Fig. 3.49 Congenital absence of the stapes suprastructure. See *arrow*

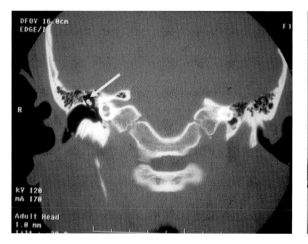

Fig. 3.47 Abnormal incus and malleus (*arrow*). Ossicular chain appears fused

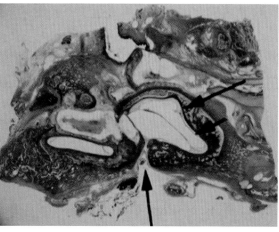

Fig. 3.50 Abnormally patent cochlear aqueduct (*single arrow*) and abnormal basal turn of the cochlea (*double arrows*)

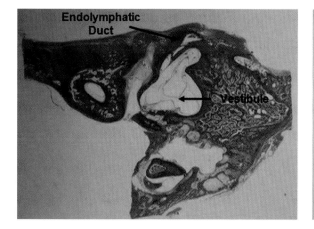

Fig. 3.48 Abnormal vestibule, wide endolymphatic duct

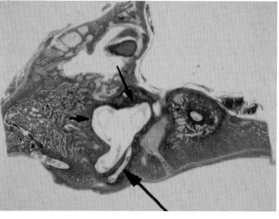

Fig. 3.51 Enlarged endolymphatic duct (*large arrow*) and abnormal semicircular canals (*smaller arrows*)

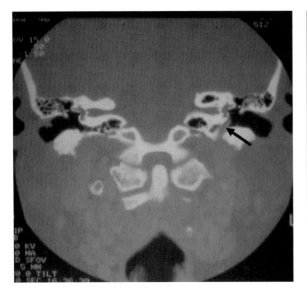

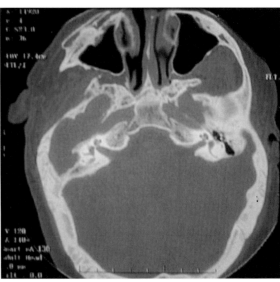

Fig. 3.52 Dehiscent internal carotid artery (*left*). See *arrow*

Fig. 3.54 Bilateral microtia and other skull base abnormalities

References

1. Baek SK, Chae SW, Jung HH (2003) Congenital internal auditory canal stenosis. J Laryngol Otol 117(10):784–787
2. Daneshi A, Farhadi M, Asghari A, Emamjomeh H, Abbasalipour P, Hasanzadeh S (2002) Three familial cases of Michel's aplasia. Otol Neurotol 23(3):346–348
3. Guirado CR (1992) Malformations of the inner auditory canal. Rev Laryngol Otol Rhinol (Bord) 113(5):419–421
4. Kitazawa K, Matsumoto M, Senda M, Honda A, Morimoto N, Kawashiro N, Imashuku S (2004) Mondini dysplasia and recurrent bacterial meningitis in a girl with relapsing Langerhans cell histiocytosis. Pediatr Blood Cancer 43(1): 85–87
5. Koyama S, Iino Y, Kaga K, Ogawa Y (1998) Facial nerve anomalies of children with congenital anomalies [Japanese]. Nippon Jibiinkoka Gakkai Kaiho 101(2):192–197
6. Paksoy Y, SEker M, Kalkan E (2004) Klippel–Feil syndrome associated with persistent trigeminal artery. Spine 29(9): E193–E196
7. Satar B, Mukherji SK, Telian SA (2003) Congenital aplasia of the semicircular canals. Otol Neurotol 24(3):437–446
8. Sennaroglu L, Saatci I (2002) A new classification for cochleovestibular malformations. Laryngoscope 112(12): 2230–2241

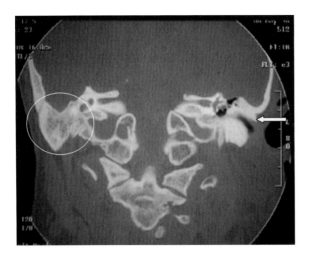

Fig. 3.53 Microtia and other skull base abnormalities. Absent external auditory canal and middle ear of the right ear (*circle*). Narrow external auditory canal of the left ear (*arrow*)

9. Sheykholeslami K, Schmerber S, Habiby Kermany M, Kaga K (2004) Vestibular-evoked myogenic potentials in three patients with large vestibular aqueduct. Hearing Res 190(1–2): 161–168

10. Triglia JM, Nicollas R, Ternier F, Cannoni M (1993) Deafness caused by malformation of the inner ear. Current contribution of x-ray computed tomography [French]. Ann Otolaryngol Chir Cervicofac 110(5):241–246

11. Tullu MS, Khanna SS, Kamat JR, Kirtane MV (2004) Mondini dysplasia and pyogenic meningitis. Indian J Pediatr 71(7):655–657

12. Zheng Y, Schachern PA, Cureoglu S, Mutlu C, Dijalilian H, Paparella MM (2002) The shortened cochlea: its classification and histopathologic features. Int J Pediat Otorhinolaryngol 63(1):29–39

13. Malekpour M, Shahidi A, Khorsandi Ashtiani MT, Motasaddi Zarandy M (2007) Novel syndrome of cataracts, retinitis pigmentosa, late onset deafness and sperm abnormalities. Am J Med Genet A 143A:1646–1652

14. Zarandy MM (2008) Transmastoid labyrinthotomy approach for cochlear implantation in a common cavity malformation. Ear Nose Throat J 87(6):E1–E3

Sudden Sensorineural Hearing Loss

4

Core Messages

> Viral, vascular, immune mediated and traumatic injury are etiologic consideration for SSNHL.

> In only 10% of SSNHL do extensive investigations establish an actual cause.

> 1–2% of SSNHL cases are identified to have a vestibular schwannoma (acoustic neuroma) on MRI scanning.

> Corticosteroid (systemic and intratympanic) therapy represents the most important treatment options.

Sudden sensorineural hearing loss (SSNHL) can be defined as an acute hearing loss of more than 20 dB of at least three contiguous audiometric frequencies occurring within 3 days or less. The hearing loss usually reaches its maximum peak within a few hours and may be accompanied by vertigo and tinnitus; the hearing loss may be unilateral or bilateral.

Idiopathic sudden sensorineural hearing loss (ISSNHL) is essentially a diagnosis of exclusion and should be entertained only after a complete search for known causes has been exhausted.

Many hypotheses have been reported to explain the etiology of SSNHL such as viral inflammation of the cochlea or cochlear nerve, vascular disease, an inner ear allergic reaction, rupture of the intralabyrinthine membranes, and autoimmune disease with the inner ear as a target organ (Figs. 4.1–4.3).

Atrophy of the organ of Corti, loss of cochlear neurons, labyrinthine fibrosis, labyrinthine hemorrhage, formation of a new bone, and degenerations of the spiral ligament, vascular stria, hair cells, dendrites, and apical spiral ganglion cells have been reported in temporal bone histopathological studies [2–4] (Figs. 4.4–4.6).

The initial evaluation for a SSNHL begins with a careful history and physical examination, looking for potential infectious causes such as acute or chronic otitis media, hematologic disorders (i.e., coagulopathies and thrombocytosis), vascular disease (i.e., thromboembolic disorders from carotid stenosis and cardiac valvular disease), autoimmune disorders, and exposure to known ototoxic medications. In some patients, further testing will be required to confirm the diagnosis. The utility of extensive blood testing in patients with no suspicious history, however, remains controversial. Unfortunately, a specific etiology for a SSNHL can be identified in only 10% of cases.

When no cause for a SSNHL is identified, one needs to still exclude retrocochlear pathology. Cerebellopontine angle lesions should always be considered in the evaluation of patients with presumed ISSNHL. Approximately 1–2% of patients with a presumed

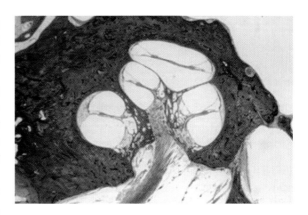

Fig. 4.1 Normal cochlea

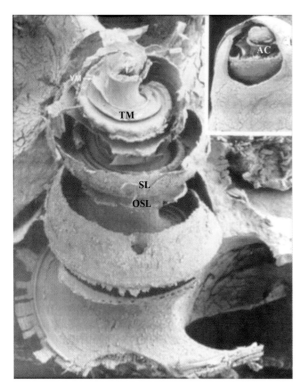

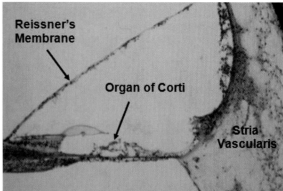

Fig. 4.4 Normal cochlea at the level of scala media

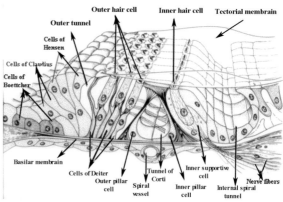

Fig. 4.2 Electromicron study of cochlea (*OHL* outer hair cells; *TM* tectorial membrane; *SV* stria vascularis)

Fig. 4.5 Schematic drawing of organ of Corti

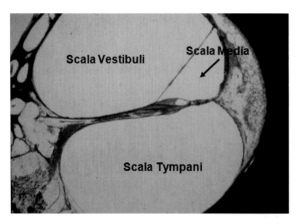

Fig. 4.3 Normal inner ear (*SV* scala vestibuli; *SM* scala media; *ST* scala tympani)

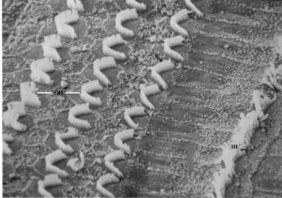

Fig. 4.6 Normal cochlea (scala media). The single row of inner hair cells and the three rows of outer hair cells are demonstrated

ISSNHL are ultimately identified to have vestibular schwannomas on contrast enhanced MRI scanning. MRI may also be able to identify other peripheral or central pathologies [1].

No discussion of an ISSNHL would be complete without discussing the controversial entity of a perilymphatic fistula. Due to the highly variable anatomy of the round window niche and membrane, it may be difficult to confirm whether a perilymphatic fistula exists especially when a mucosal web or fibrous tissue appears over the round window niche (Figs. 4.7–4.9).

Vascular compromise of the inner ear as a cause of SSNHL has been documented in patients undergoing oral anticoagulant therapy. It is conceivable that oral anticoagulants influence the viscosity of the plasma which in return interferes with the microcirculation in the inner ear [5].

When no identifiable cause is found, several treatment methods can be used to treat a SSNHL either alone or in combination. At the present time, however, there is no universally accepted treatment for acute SSNHL. In fact, it is difficult to know within the confines of evidence-based medicine, whether any treatment will influence the natural history of this condition.

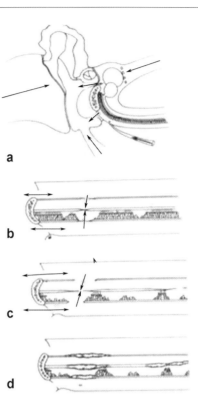

Fig. 4.9 Schematic diagram demonstrating both perilymphatic and intracochlear fistulae formation. **a** implosive and explosive routes, **b** intracochlear injury to hair cells and basilar membrane, **c** intracochlear membrane ruptures, **d** healing of intracochlear membrane ruptures

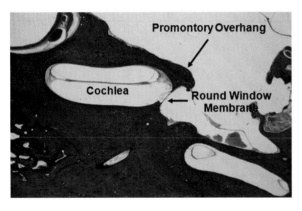

Fig. 4.7 Normal appearance of the round window

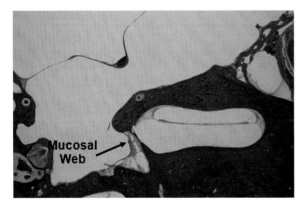

Fig. 4.8 Mucosal web in the round window

The majority of treatments are based on the two common theories of its etiology: circulatory disturbance and inflammatory reaction (mostly viral) (Figs. 4.10 and 4.11).

Numerous treatments have been proposed to improve the cochlear blood flow (CBF) by vasodilation (histamine, papaverine, verapamil, and carbon dioxide) or by decreasing the blood viscosity (dextran and papaverine) and by reducing any accompanying inflammatory reaction [2, 5].

Corticosteroids (systemic and intratympanic) are widely used in the treatment of a sudden hearing loss. The specific action of steroids is unknown, but they may be beneficial in infectious, inflammatory, and immune-mediated conditions. The use of antiviral treatments in the management of SSNHL remains controversial. One typical treatment regimen where every potential cause is covered includes a "shotgun" regimen of low molecular weight dextran, histamine,

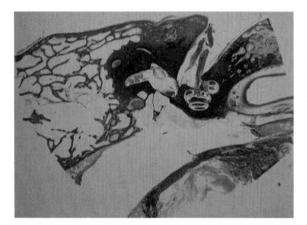

Fig. 4.10 Cochlear hemorrhage with sudden hearing loss

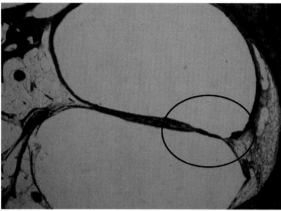

Fig. 4.12 Severe sensorineural deafness that occurred as the result of a lightening stike to an unfortunate individual. Note the complete loss of the organ of Corti as demonstrated by the circle

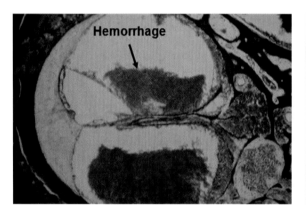

Fig. 4.11 Cochlear hemorrhage with sudden hearing loss. Note that hemorrhage appears to involve the perilymphatic space primarily

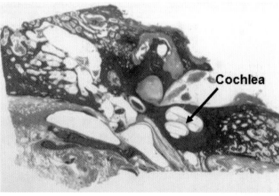

Fig. 4.13 Skull base osteomyelitis resulting in suppurative labrynthitis

hypaque, diuretics, steroids, vasodilators, and carbogen inhalation [2].

The prognosis is highly variable and depends on the time of presentation from when the hearing loss occurred, the severity of the hearing loss, the probable cause, and the presence of other factors such as vertigo and tinnitus and the audiometric configuration of the hearing loss (a low frequency loss appears to have a more favorable prognosis) [1, 4] (Figs. 4.12–4.15).

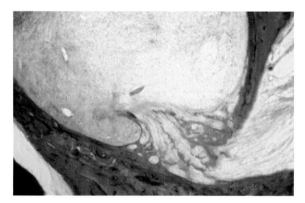

Fig. 4.14 Suppurative labyrinthitis associated with sudden sensorineural hearing loss

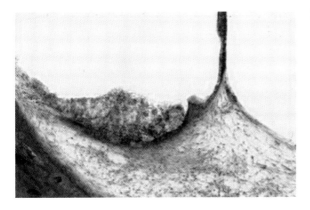

Fig. 4.15 Suppurative cochleitis affecting scala media and stria vascularis

References

1. Aarnisalo AA, Suoranta H, Ylikoski J (2004) Magnetic resonance imaging findings in the auditory pathway of patients with sudden deafness. Otol Neurotol 25(3):245–249
2. Haberkamp TJ, Tanyeri HM (1999) Management of idiopathic sudden sensorineural hearing loss. Am J Otol 20(5): 587–592; discussion 593–595
3. Ito S, Fuse T, Yokota M, Watanabe T, Inamura K, Gon S, Aoyagi M (2002) Prognosis is predicted by early hearing improvement in patients with idiopathic sudden sensorineural hearing loss. Clin Otolaryngol Allied Sci 27(6):501–504
4. Koc A, Sanisoglu O (2003) Sudden sensorineural hearing loss: literature survey on recent studies. J Otolaryngol 32(5):308–313
5. Mierzwa K, Schneider G, Muller A (2004) Sudden sensorineural hearing loss during oral anticoagulant therapy. J Laryngol Otol 118(11):872–876

Trauma to the Inner Ear

5

Core Messages

> Temporal bone fractures are best classified as "otic capsule-sparing" or "otic capsule-violating".

> Otic capsule-violating fractures are more likely to be associated with facial paralysis, CSF leakage, a profound sensorineural hearing loss, vertigo and an intracranial hemorrhage.

> A high resolution CT scan is the investigation of choice for fracture localization.

> Following skull fracture patients continue to be at greater risk for meningitis.

Temporal bone (TB) fractures are seen in 6–8% of patients following severe head trauma and in 10–22% of patients with skull fractures. The direction, magnitude, and anatomic location of the traumatic force as well as the bony density of the skull help determine the orientation of the fracture plane.

TB fractures are classically divided into longitudinal fractures, transverse fractures, and mixed fractures; the designation indicating the fracture line relative to the long axis of the petrous bone. While being anatomically useful, these classifications are not always helpful in predicting the severity of clinical symptoms and signs. A classification involving "otic capsule sparing" vs. "otic capsule violating" fractures is probably more specific.

This classification system that emphasizes violation or lack of violation of the otic capsule seems to offer the advantage of radiographic utility and stratification of clinical severity (Figs. 5.1–5.4).

Otic capsule violating fractures are relatively rare. Compared to otic capsule-sparing fractures they are approximately two and four times more likely to develop a facial paralysis and CSF leak, respectively, and seven times more likely to experience profound hearing loss. They are more likely as well to sustain intracranial complications including subarachnoid hemorrhage and epidural hematoma [2, 6].

Capsule-violating fractures frequently damage the structures within or coursing through the TB, leading to facial paralysis, cerebrospinal fluid fistula, sensorineural and/or conductive hearing loss, and vertigo [1, 3, 6] (Figs. 5.5–5.7).

It is recommended that all patients, following a TB fracture, should undergo otological assessment as well as facial nerve evaluation. This will facilitate the early detection and subsequent treatment of potentially

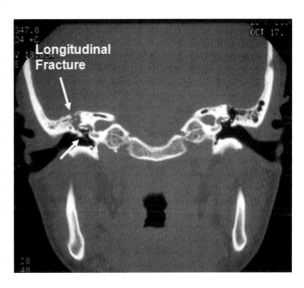

Fig. 5.1 Incus dislocation (see *arrow*) into the external auditory canal following a longitudinal fracture of the temporal bone

M. M. Zarandy and J. Rutka, *Diseases of the Inner Ear*
DOI: 10.1007/978-3-642-05058-9_5, © Springer-Verlag Berlin Heidelberg 2010

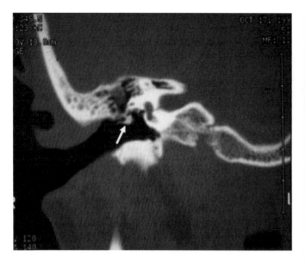

Fig. 5.2 Incus dislocation into the external auditory canal (Same patient as in Fig. 5.1). See *arrow*

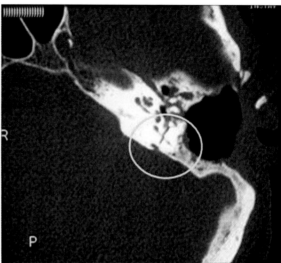

Fig. 5.5 Axial CT scan of the temporal bone demonstrating transverse fracture (otic capsule-violating fracture). See *circle*

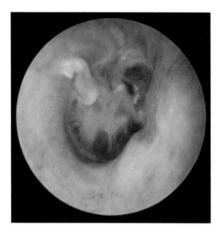

Fig. 5.3 Dislocation of incus into ear canal following longitudinal fracture (Same patient as in Fig. 5.1)

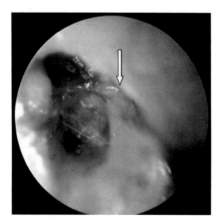

Fig. 5.4 Longitudinal fracture of the temporal bone demonstrating step deformity in ear canal. See *arrow*

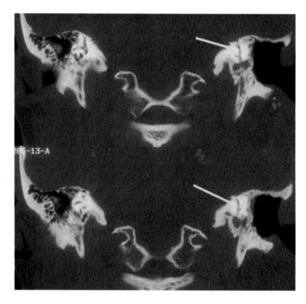

Fig. 5.6 Coronal CT scan demonstrating transverse fractures through the otic capsule. See *arrow*

correctable middle ear and facial nerve injury [4]. However, this may prove difficult in an unconscious patient. Nevertheless, it has been established that the earlier the facial nerve decompression, the more beneficial the procedure is for the recovery of the facial nerve function [3].

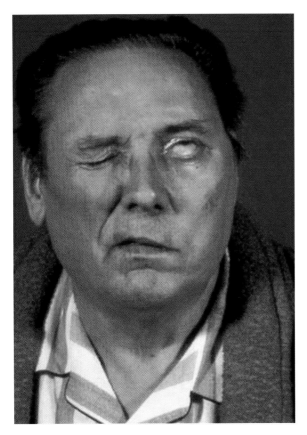

Fig. 5.7 Left facial paralysis resulting from a fracture of the temporal bone

This is especially true when bone fragments in the fracture lines compress the facial nerve preventing axonal regrowth.

Despite clinical healing of the fracture line following skull fracture, patients continue to remain at a higher risk for meningitis throughout life [6].

Thin-section, high-resolution computed tomography (CT) scan is the procedure of choice for confirming a TB fracture. As an investigation, it can help delineate the fracture lines, differentiate between an otic capsule sparing and violating fracture and can provide information regarding a traumatic dislocation of the ossicular chain. High-resolution CT scan can additionally show the entire course of the facial nerve in the coronal and axial sections. Fracture fragments or evidence of localized expansion indicate the presence of an intraneural hematoma or edema.

MRI is generally recommended for patients suspected of having sustained an intracranial complication, due to its greater ability to delineate parenchymal abnormalities and extracerebral collections. It can also be useful in confirming the disruption of the tegmen tympani and to distinguish blood from the edematous mucosa in the mastoid air cells and the CSF within the middle ear or the mastoid air cells.

Patients with a sensorineural hearing loss following trauma who have no obvious fracture on a CT scan are often diagnosed as having a "labyrinthine concussion." MRI with gadolinium may play an important role in confirming the diagnosis in such cases [2, 3, 6].

Fractures through the endochondral part of the cochlear capsule do not heal by callus formation but persist as a layer of fibrous tissue. This is possibly because endochondral bone is mature at birth and does not undergo remodeling throughout life. While the presence of microfractures involving otic capsule and their significance remains uncertain, they are not an infrequent finding in TB histopathology (Figs. 5.8–5.11).

Despite the best intention of the health care providers, inadvertent injury to the inner ear can occur as a result of iatrogenic injury. Great care should be taken during surgery to prevent such an injury and during procedures performed in out patient settings [5] (Figs. 5.12–5.16).

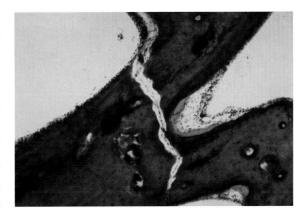

Fig. 5.8 Microfracture (cochlea to internal auditory canal). The presence of mature fibrous tissue in the fracture site makes it unlikely to be an artifact or post mortem finding

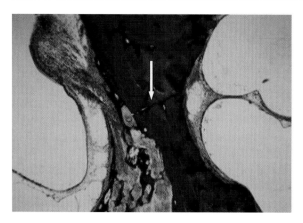

Fig. 5.9 Microfracture of the otic capsule. See *arrow*

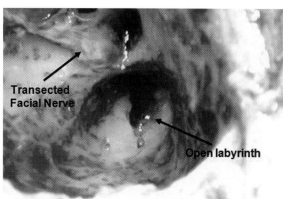

Fig. 5.12 Iatrogenic injury to the labyrinth and facial nerve during mastoid surgery for cholesteatoma. See *arrows*

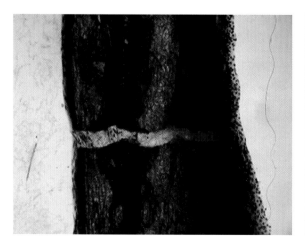

Fig. 5.10 Microfracture of the otic capsule

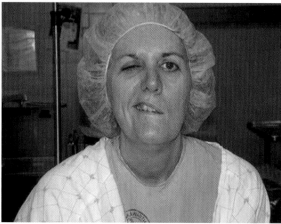

Fig. 5.13 Left facial nerve paralysis following mechanical injury to the inner ear following syringing

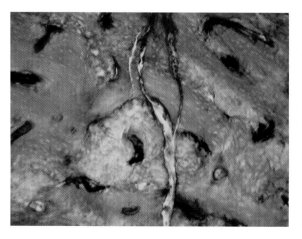

Fig. 5.11 Microfracture of the otic capsule. Note the fibrous healing of the fracture site in endochondral derived bone

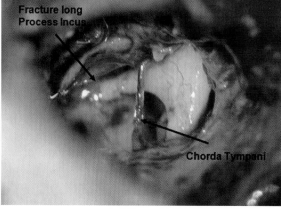

Fig. 5.14 Dislocation and fracture of the long process of incus with trauma to stapes. Facial nerve sustained a crush injury in its horizontal segment (Same patient as in Fig. 5.13)

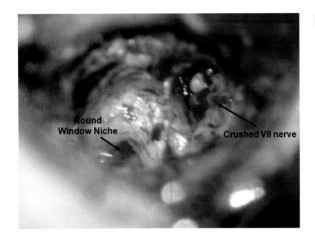

Fig. 5.15 Crush injury to facial nerve and injury to stapes (Same patient as in Fig. 5.10)

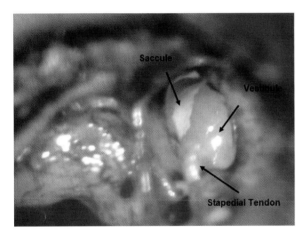

Fig. 5.16 Open vestibule following removal of dislocated stapes which had caused a perilymphatic fistula. Note the stapedial tendon and the saccule inside the vestibule

References

1. Dahiya R, Keller JD, Litofsky NS, Bankey PE, Bonassar LJ, Megerian CA (1999) Temporal bone fractures: otic capsule sparing versus otic capsule violating clinical and radiographic considerations. J Trauma 47(6):1079–1083
2. Gross M, Yaacov AB, Eliashar R (2003) Cochlear involvement in a temporal bone fracture. Otol Neurotol 24(6): 958–959
3. Kinoshita T, Ishii K, Okitsu T, Okudera T, Ogawa T (2001) Facial nerve palsy: evaluation by contrast-enhanced MR imaging. Clin Radiol 56(11):926–932
4. Lancaster JL, Alderson DJ, Curley JW (1999) Otological complications following basal skull fractures. J R Coll Surg Edinb 44(2):87–90
5. Motasaddi Zarandy. Mahdi Malekpour (2007) Two cochlear implant: halving the number of recipients. Lancet 370:1686
6. Sudhoff H, Linthicum FH Jr (2003) Temporal bone fracture and latent meningitis: temporal bone histopathology study of the month. Otol Neurotol 24(3):521–522

Otosclerosis

Core Messages

> Otosclerosis is unique to the human otic capsule. It is an autosommal dominant genetic disorder with incomplete clinical penetrance.

> Progressive conductive hearing loss from stapes fixation arises from the dual pathologic processes of otospongiosis and otosclerosis.

> Primary cochlear otosclerosis is relatively rare.

> Stapes surgery or fitting of a hearing aid can rehabilitate the hearing loss.

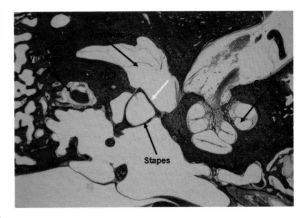

Fig. 6.1 Normal footplate (see *arrow*)

Otosclerosis is the most common primary osseous lesion of the temporal bone. It is a disease of unknown etiology with a strong genetic predisposition that primarily affects the endochondral derived bone of the otic capsule in the region of the stapes footplate. New immature bone formation (termed otospongiosis) tends to mechanically interfere with the movement of the stapes which in turn leads to a progressive conductive hearing loss. Additionally, tinnitus is often present. The disease process may be accelerated in pregnancy suggesting a hormonal influence. Less frequent involvement of other parts of the otic capsule and the underlying inner ear structures is thought to be responsible for the sensorineural hearing loss and any accompanying dizziness/imbalance [2] (Figs. 6.1–6.5).

The etiology of otosclerosis remains elusive. The role of collagen type 2, genetic factors, and measles virus infection as causal factors is often mentioned. From an epidemiological point of view, the disease

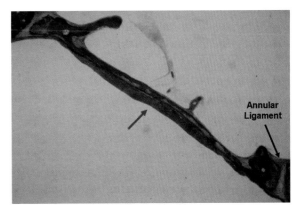

Fig. 6.2 Normal footplate. See *arrow*. Note the annular ligament

has an autosomal dominant mode of inheritance with incomplete penetrance.

It has been reported that the incidence of clinical otosclerosis has diminished in recent years from the addition of fluoride to the drinking water. Others have suggested that the administration of measles vaccination

M. M. Zarandy and J. Rutka, *Diseases of the Inner Ear*
DOI: 10.1007/978-3-642-05058-9_6, © Springer-Verlag Berlin Heidelberg 2010

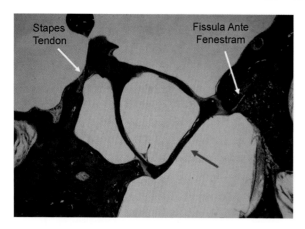

Fig. 6.3 Normal stapes. The fissula ante fenestram (a suspected cartilaginous rest) in the otic capsule is often suspected as the initial site for otosclerosis involvement of the otic capsule. See *longer white arrow. Red arrow* demonstrates the stapes footplate

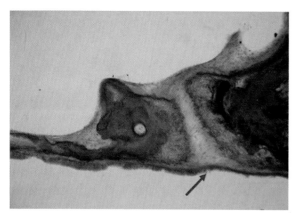

Fig. 6.4 Normal annular ligament (see *red arrow*)

By definition, "clinical" otosclerosis implies that the otosclerotic lesion(s) has typically resulted in stapes fixation causing a conductive hearing loss. "Histological" otosclerosis means that one or more foci of otosclerosis can be found in the otic capsule without causing stapes fixation. The term "Cochlear" otosclerosis is used when histological otosclerosis has replaced some part of the endosteal layer of the bone of cochlea that not infrequently results in a sensorineural hearing loss." In any individual, all three types of otosclerosis may be present (Figs. 6.5–6.7).

The characteristic histological findings in otosclerosis occur only in the otic capsule. Otosclerosis occurs in two phases: an early active phase (otospongiotic stage)

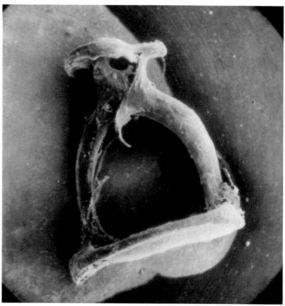

Fig. 6.5 Normal stapes

to children has altered the clinical presentation of otosclerosis. Niedermeyer from Germany reported that the increase in the average age of patients having primary stapes surgery from 1978 to 1999 strongly supported the effect of measles vaccination in decreasing the incidence of otosclerosis. A viral influence, however, is not supported by significant racial differences in the disease [1, 4].

Otosclerosis appears to be more common in caucasians than other races. If searched for, it is histologically present at autopsy in approximately 10% of Caucasians. Less than 1/400, however, will demonstrate a clinical evidence of the disease.

Clinical otosclerosis affects women approximately twice as often as men. As previously mentioned, it may be exacerbated by pregnancy and puberty.

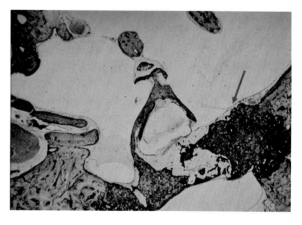

Fig. 6.6 Otosclerotic foci involving the footplate. See *red arrow*

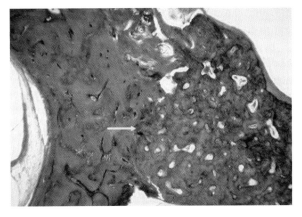

Fig. 6.7 Cochlear otosclerosis. Note the immature "sponge-like" bone (otospongiosus) of the otosclerotic foci. Junction of the normal vs. otosclerotic bone marked by *yellow arrow*

during which bone resorption occurs, and a later inactive phase (sclerotic stage).

In the active phase, osteolytic lesions appear in the endochondral layer of the otic capsule, resulting in a disorganized formation of woven bone with marrow spaces containing osteoblasts, osteocytes, connective tissue, and blood vessels. The vacuolated areas in the foci are filled with a soft tissue and are much less dense than the normal labyrinthine bone. In these areas, there seems to be a predominance of osteoclasts (lacunae of Howship), giant cells, fibroblasts, and proliferating endothelial cells in the foci (Fig. 6.8).

Over a period of time, the foci undergo a decrease in their cellularity, an obliteration of the blood vessels, remineralization, and reorganization to a sclerotic lamellar bone. Both the phases of the process may be simultaneously present.

Metabolic activity within the otosclerotic focus is variable and most cases of otosclerosis show evidence of mixed activity with one level of activity usually predominating. The otosclerotic process may become quiescent at any time or may subsequently become reactivated in a previously quiescent area.

In otosclerosis, three major patterns of involvement are discussed: the fenestral type, the cochlear type, and the mixed type. In the fenestral type, the focus is located initially at the oval window near the fissula ante fenestram, with the possible involvement of the stapes footplate (Figs. 6.9–6.12).

The cochlear type has typical irregular and discontinuous hypodensities caused by demineralization in the endochondral bone of the otic capsule.

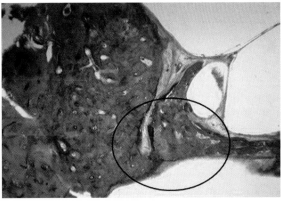

Fig. 6.9 Otosclerosis involving the stapes footplate as demonstrated by a *circle*

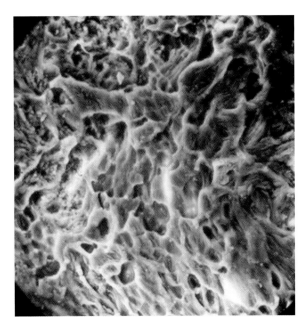

Fig. 6.8 Otosclerosis on electron microscopy

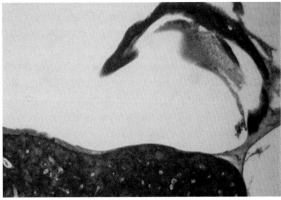

Fig. 6.10 Otosclerosis involving the footplate

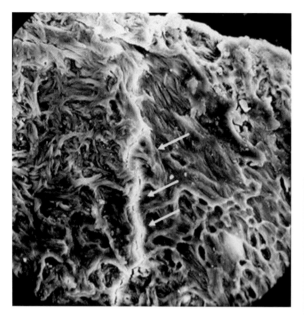

Fig. 6.11 Demarcation of the normal vs. otosclerotic bone. See *arrows*

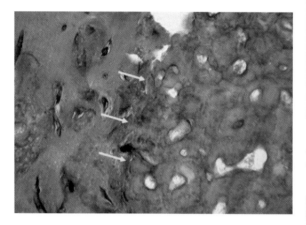

Fig. 6.12 The junction between the normal and otosclerotic bone (See *arrows*)

In the mixed type, there is involvement of the pericochlear otic capsule together with stapes footplate involvement [3, 5].

The diagnosis of otosclerosis is the one that requires the exclusion of other causes for hearing loss and is based on the clinical findings, audiometric testing (and tympanometry with stapedial reflex testing) especially when a strong family history is present. High resolution CT of the temporal bones may be helpful in confirming the cochlear involvement.

In high-resolution CT, the spongiotic phase of the cochlear type presents as areas of demineralization in

the otic capsule surrounding the cochlea (so-called fourth coil or double-ring sign) [7].

In magnetic resonance imaging (MRI), enhancement of the otic capsule has been established in patients with active otosclerosis. The enhancement is presumably caused by the pooling of contrast medium in the blood vessels and lacunae of the otospongiotic (active) foci.

Stapedectomy surgery in carefully selected cases may help to improve the hearing (Figs. 6.13–6.16).

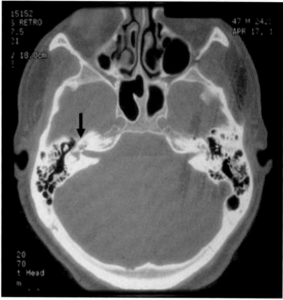

Fig. 6.13 High resolution CT scan demonstrating significant demineralization around the cochlea (the so-called fourth coil or signet ring sign). See *black arrow*

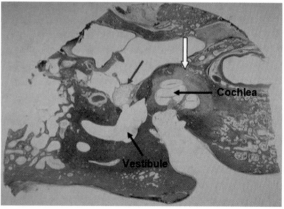

Fig. 6.14 Axial cross-section of the temporal bone demonstrating the presence of a fat wire prosthesis. See *red arrow* Cochlear otosclerosis is suspected as well by the significant demineralization of the bone surrounding the cochlea. See *arrow*

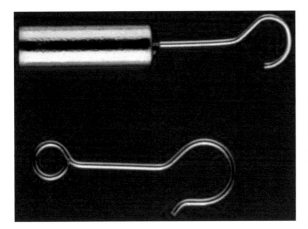

Fig. 6.15 Metallic stapes piston prosthesis for the surgical correction of hearing loss in stapedectomy surgery

The differential diagnosis for otosclerosis includes osteogenesis imperfecta, labyrinthitis ossificans, and Paget's disease [6, 7] (Figs. 6.17–6.20).

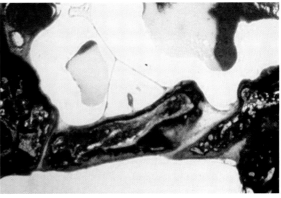

Fig. 6.17 Bony change in osteogenesis imperfecta involving the stapes footplate. This inherited condition may cause a conductive hearing loss similar to otosclerosis in many ways. Stapedectomy surgery in carefully selected cases may help to improve the hearing

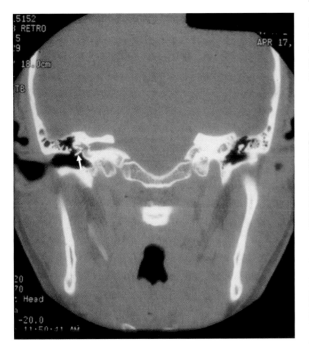

Fig. 6.16 CT scan demonstrating the stapes prosthesis in the right ear. See *arrow*

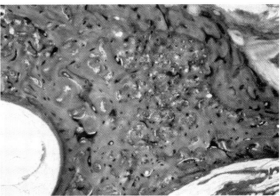

Fig. 6.18 Histopathology of Paget's disease. While unlikely to cause a conductive hearing loss, it is a part of the differential diagnosis

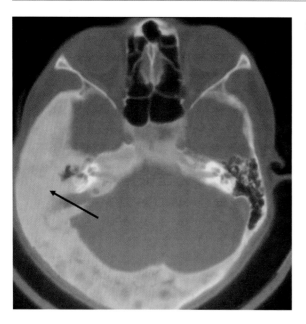

Fig. 6.19 Fibrous dysplasia may involve the middle ear and result in a conductive hearing loss. *Black arrow* demonstrates the "ground glass" appearance of bone in fibrous dysplasia

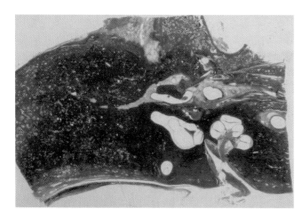

Fig. 6.20 Osteopetrosis or marble bone disease. Inherited disorder that results in the formation of a hard compact, yet paradoxically brittle bone with the replacement of bone marrow. Patients are prone to pathological fractures, anemia, and facial paralysis

References

1. Hawke M, John AF (1987) Diseases of the ear, clinical and pathologic aspects. Gower, New York
2. Karosi T, Konya J, Szabo LZ, Sziklai I (2004) Measles virus prevalence in otosclerotic stapes footplate samples. Otol Neurotol 25(4):451–456
3. Mahfudz Z, Lokman S (2004) Outcome of stapes surgery for otosclerosis. Med J Malaysia 59(2):171–176
4. Menger DJ, Tange RA (2003) The aetiology of otosclerosis: a review of the literature. Clin Otolaryngol Allied Sci 28(2): 112–120
5. Meyer TA, Lambert PR (2004) Primary and revision stapedectomy in elderly patients. Curr Opin Otolaryngol Head Neck Surg 12(5):387–392
6. Nelson EG, Hinojosa R (2004) Questioning the relationship between cochlear otosclerosis and sensorineural hearing loss: a quantitative evaluation of cochlear structures in cases of otosclerosis and review of the literature [see comment]. Laryngoscope 114(7):1214–1230
7. Nowe V, Verstreken M, Wuyts FL, Van de Heyning P, De Schepper AM, Parizel PM (2004) Enhancement of the otic capsule in active retrofenestral otosclerosis [Case Reports. Journal Article]. Otol Neurotol 25(4):633–634

Presbycusis

Core Messages

> Presbycusis and noise-induced hearing loss (NIHL) are the leading cause for sensorineural hearing loss in today's society.

> Cochlear degeneration in presbycusis is caused by complex genetic determinants influenced by environmental noise exposure.

> While primarily cochlear, changes in presbycusis can involve all parts of the auditory system.

> No cure for presbycusis exists. Concomitant noise induced hearing loss can be prevented. Aural rehabilitation can provided when hearing is sufficiently impaired.

Hearing thresholds not infrequently worsen with age and results in a progressive hearing loss known as presbycusis.

Presbycusis represents the most common cause of sensorineural hearing loss (SNHL) in today's society. Audiometry usually demonstrates a bilateral (typically high frequency) symmetrical SNHL with absent or partial recruitment (Figs. 7.1–7.3).

In susceptible individuals, the effects of presbycusis are first apparent in early middle age (often starting around age 40). The hearing loss worsens progressively as years pass.

Presbycusis definitely affects an individual's quality of life as he or she age. As the elderly proportion of the population appears to be increasing, it would not be unreasonable to expect an increase in the incidence of presbycusis in future.

Presbycusis is usually caused by a cochlear degeneration which is most pronounced in the basal cochlear coil. The most common audiometric configuration is that of a gently-sloping audiogram, initially, above all affecting the higher frequencies.

The etiology of presbycusis remains uncertain. However, it would appear that a complex genetic cause is most likely, that may be influenced by the environmental noise exposure throughout an individual's lifespan.

Based on the correlations between the audiometric configurations and histological findings gathered from postmortem examinations, Schuknecht proposed that four types of presbycusis can be identified, namely: sensorineural, neural, strial, and cochlear conductive [3] (Figs. 7.4 and 7.5).

Pathological appearances in presbycusis also vary. Degenerative changes vary in their site of involvement and extent. They are not limited necessarily to the cochlear structures, but can also be found in all parts of the auditory system [2].

The most prominent histopathological change within the inner ear is a decrease in the population of the spiral ganglion (SG) cells. Diffuse senile atrophy is also often seen in the organ of Corti and the stria vascularis (Figs. 7.6 and 7.7).

Ultrastructural analysis reveals the degeneration of inner ear hair cells and supporting cells especially in the basal turn of the cochlea. There are marked degenerative changes of the remaining neural fibers as well. These changes include a decrease in the number of synapses at the base of the hair cells, accumulation of cellular debris within the spiral bundles, abnormalities of the dendritic fibers and their sheaths in the osseous spiral lamina, and degenerative changes in the SG cells and axons. In addition, there is a marked thickening of the basilar membrane

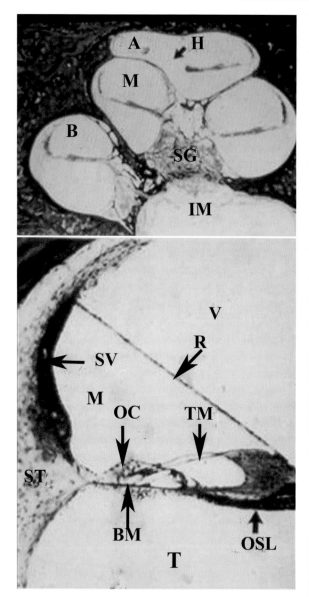

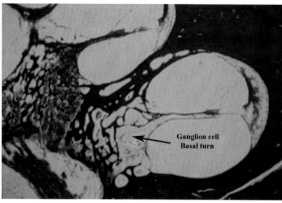

Fig. 7.2 Presbycusis (reduction of ganglion cells noted). See *arrow*

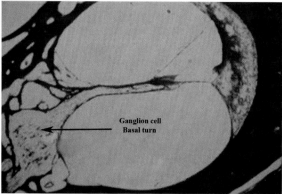

Fig. 7.3 Presbycusis (higher magnification). See *arrow*

Fig. 7.1 Normal cochlea (*R* Reissner's membrane; *OSL* osseous spiral lamina; *SL* spiral ligament; *BM* basilar membrane; *OC* outer cells; *TM* tectorial membrane; *SV* stria vascularis; *T* scala tympani; *V* scala vestibule; *M* scala media; *B* basal turn; *M* middle turn; *A* apical turn; *SG* spiral ganglion; *IM* internal auditory meatus)

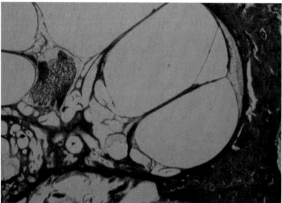

Fig. 7.4 Presbycusis, neural type

(BM) in the basal turn which consists of an increased number of fibrils and an accumulation of amorphous osmophilic material in the BM. These findings support the concept that mechanical alterations may occur in presbycusis of the basal turn [8] (Figs. 7.8 and 7.9).

Efforts to improve communication in old age are important because hearing loss is often combined with other handicaps, such as dementia, immobility, and poor

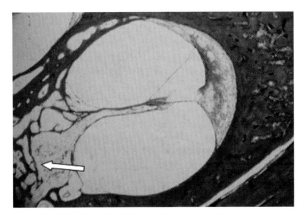

Fig. 7.5 Presbycusis, absent ganglion cell of basal turn. See *arrow*

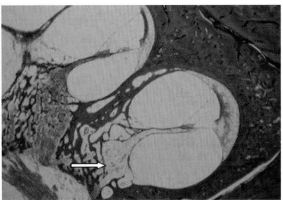

Fig. 7.8 Presbycusis, neural type, absent ganglion cell of basal turn. See *arrow*

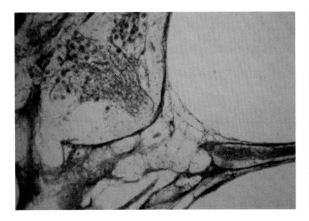

Fig. 7.6 Spiral ganglion cells

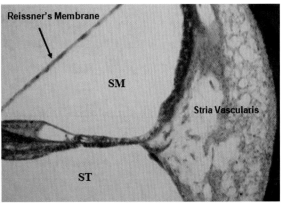

Fig. 7.9 Presbycusis due to strial atrophy (*ST* scala tympani; *SM* scala media)

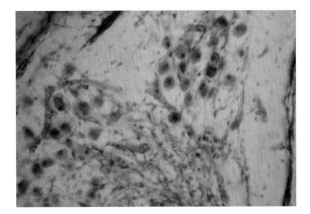

Fig. 7.7 Spiral ganglion cells (Higher magnification)

vision. The synergistic effects of multiple handicaps can be extensive and should not be overlooked [4–6].

To date, there are only two possible treatments for presbycusis:

1. Prevention: Prevention is a concept which is both challenging and problematic. The most important preventive measure requires noise reduction and hearing protection if exposed to loud noise potentially injurious to hearing. This must start early in life and not shortly before retirement. Considerable gains can be achieved with respect to resources (both human and economical) through rehabilitation and suitable preventive measures especially in industry [7].
2. Fitting of an appropriate hearing aid.

It is important to realize that hearing usually decreases with age in most, but not all individuals. Some older people may appear to be completely normal audiometrically, despite complaints of hearing loss. It is presumed deficits not only occur within the inner ear, but also within central auditory pathways [1].

References

1. Hesse G (2004) Hearing aids in the elderly. Why is the accommodation so difficult? [German]. HNO 52(4): 321–328
2. Nadol JB Jr (1979) Electron microscopic findings in presbycusic degeneration of the basal turn of the human cochlea. Otolaryngol Head Neck Surg 87(6):818–836
3. Pata YS, Akbas Y, Unal M, Duce MN, Akbas T, Micozkadioglu D (2004) The relationship between presbycusis and mastoid pneumatization. Yonsei Med J 45(1): 68–72
4. Rosenhall U (2001) Presbyacusis–hearing loss in old age [Swedish]. Lakartidningen 98(23):2802–2806
5. Scholtz AW, Kammen-Jolly K, Felder E, Hussl B, Rask-Andersen H, Schrott-Fischer A (2001) Selective aspects of human pathology in high-tone hearing loss of the aging inner ear. Hear Res 157(1–2):77–86
6. Schuknecht HF, Gacek MR (1993) Cochlear pathology in presbycusis. Ann Otol Rhinol Laryngol 102:1–16
7. Schultz-Coulon HJ (1985) Hearing in advanced age: critical view of so-called presbycusis [German]. HNO 33(1):2–10
8. Suga F, Lindsay JR (1976) Histopathological observations of presbycusis. Ann Otol Rhinol Laryngol 85(2 pt1): 169–184

Ménière's Syndrome

8

Core Messages

> Ménière's syndrome is defined by spontaneous attacks of episodic vertigo, fluctuant sensorineural hearing loss, tinnitus and a sense of aural pressure in an affected ear.

> When idiopathic Ménière's syndrome is referred to as Ménière's disease.

> Endolymphatic hydrops is the most consistent pathologic change at autopsy.

> No cure exists. A large number of medical and surgical treatments are available.

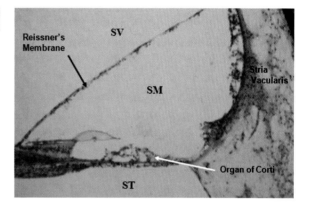

Fig. 8.1 Normal cochlea (*SV* scala vestibule; *SM* scala media; *ST* scala tympani)

Ménière's syndrome is an inner-ear disorder marked by spontaneous attacks of vertigo, fluctuating sensorineural hearing loss, aural fullness, and tinnitus [6].

The actual onset of vertigo is usually sudden and severe, often associated with nausea and vomiting. The vertigo usually lasts for a few hours, not infrequently followed by hours of unsteadiness. The attacks may awaken the patient from sleep [6].

In the early stages of the disease, hearing loss is usually found in the lower frequencies and tends to recover in between attacks. Over time, however, it becomes permanent and extends to involve all frequencies. In general, the sensorineural hearing loss in Ménière's disease is typically fluctuating and progressive.

When the syndrome is idiopathic and not attributable to a specifically identified cause, it is referred to as Ménière's disease. A slight female to male preponderance (1.3:1) has been observed in its prevalence (Fig. 8.1).

The peak incidence for Ménière's disease appears in the 40–60-year age-group. Unilateral involvement initially is typical. Subsequent involvement of the contralateral ear has been reported in up to 50% over the course of an individual's lifetime. Dilation of the membranous labyrinth, termed as endolymphatic hydrops is considered to be the pathophysiologic cause. Accordingly, Ménière's disease has been postulated to be a disorder of the intralabyrinthine fluid dynamics.

Endolymphatic hydrops, histologically, is most consistently found in the cochlea and saccule in Ménière's disease. It is typified by the ballooning of the Reissner's membrane into the scala vestibuli of the cochlea and by the distention of the saccule. Changes in the utricle and semicircular canals can be seen but are generally less dramatic. Proteinaceous staining in the scala media is not infrequently identified, although its significance still remains to be determined [1, 8].

Ruptures in Reissner's membrane or in the walls of the saccule and utricle are thought to be significant in

M. M. Zarandy and J. Rutka, *Diseases of the Inner Ear*
DOI: 10.1007/978-3-642-05058-9_8, © Springer-Verlag Berlin Heidelberg 2010

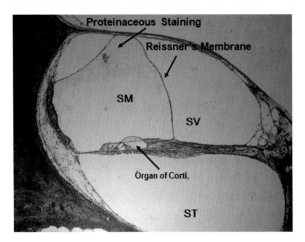

Fig. 8.2 Hydrops in Ménière's disease. Note the proteinaceous staining at the top of the scala media additionally (*SM* scala media; *SV* scala vestibule; *ST* scala tympani)

the pathophysiology of Ménière's disease. Ruptures occur more frequently in Reissner's membrane than in vestibular membranes [8] (Fig. 8.2).

Autoimmune processes have also been implicated as etiologic factors. For example, elevated antibodies directed against type II collagen have been demonstrated in some Ménière's patients. Some patients have also been noted to have abnormal levels of immune complexes and circulating complement. Viral infection causing damage to the endolymphatic sac and duct is yet another suggested cause for Ménière's disease.

Imaging studies of patients with Ménière's disease have identified abnormalities of the endolymphatic drainage system. Such studies suggest hypoplasia of the endolymphatic sac and duct. Magnetic resonance imaging (MRI) reveals that patients with Ménière's disease may have smaller and shorter endolymph drainage systems. Enhancement of the endolymphatic sac has also been seen on gadolinium-enhanced images. This has been interpreted by some as inflammation of the sac in these patients.

Although endolymphatic hydrops can only be conclusively proven upon necropsy on histopathologic examination, The American Academy of Otolaryngology – Head and Neck Surgery (AAO-HNS) has recommended guidelines for making a diagnosis of "a definite" Ménière's disease. This includes two or more spontaneous episodes of vertigo each lasting for 20 min or longer, hearing loss documented by

audiograms on at least one occasion, tinnitus or aural fullness in the affected ear upon the exclusion of other causes (specifically with MRI). It is important to realize that the classic symptoms necessary for diagnosis may not always be present simultaneously or in the same pattern, particularly in the early phases of the disease.

A caloric reduction in the affected ear has been observed in 48–74% of patients with Ménière's disease. Absent caloric responses in the affected ear are identified in 6–11% of patients. Electrocochleography (ECoG) has also been used in the diagnosis of Ménière's disease. The ratio of the summating potential (SP) to the action potential (AP) (or SP/AP ratio) has been reported to be increased in patients with Ménière's disease. The accuracy of ECoG in the diagnosis of Ménière's disease, however, has been controversial. The measurement of low-frequency modulated distorsion product otoacoustic emissions (DPOAEs) is reported to be a new tool for the diagnosis and clinical monitoring of endolymphatic hydrops and in evaluating the effectiveness of the therapeutic methods [2, 5, 7].

At present, there is no universal cure for Ménière's disease. Current therapy is directed at the reduction of the associated symptoms (Fig. 8.3).

Medical regimens include salt restriction, diuretics, and vasodilators (i.e., betahistine). Steroids administered orally or through intratympanic injection have also been used in the management of Ménière's disease. Intratympanic aminoglycoside vestibular ablation/attentuation has been especially effective in controlling the vertigo caused by Ménière's disease [3, 4].

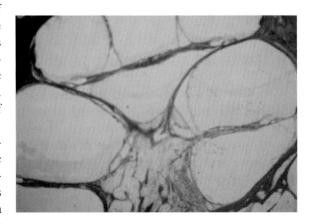

Fig. 8.3 Cross section of the human cochlea demonstrating endolymphatic hydrops. Note the proteinaceous staining within the inner ear as well

In patients in whom vertigo persists despite a trial of optimal medical therapy, other forms of treatment are indicated. Surgical procedures performed on the endolymphatic sac are designed to either decompress the sac or to drain the endolymph. Selective vestibular neurectomy performed via a middle cranial fossa or posterior cranial fossa approach has also been used to achieve control of the vertigo in over 90% of patients whose vertigo had proven intractable and refractive to medical therapy. Labyrinthectomy in selected cases may also be effective but precludes any hearing preservation.

References

1. Andrews JC (2004) Intralabyrinthine fluid dynamics: Meniere disease. Curr Opin Otolaryngol Head Neck Surg 12(5):408–412

2. Ghosh S, Gupta AK, Mann SS (2002) Can electrocochleography in Meniere's disease be noninvasive. J Otolaryngol 31(6):371–375

3. Gossow-Muller-Hohenstein E, Hirschfelder A, Scholz G, Mrowinski D (2003) Aural fullness and endolymphatic hydrops. Laryngorhinootologie [German] 82(2):97–101

4. Hillman TM, Arriaga MA, Chen DA (2003) Intratympanic steroids: do they acutely improve hearing in cases of cochlear hydrops? Laryngoscope 113(11):1903–1907

5. Magliulo G, Cianfrone G, Gagliardi M, Cuiuli G, D'Amico R (2004) Vestibular evoked myogenic potentials and distortion-product otoacoustic emissions combined with glycerol testing in endolymphatic hydrops: their value in early diagnosis. Ann Otol Rhinol Laryngol 113(12):1000–1005

6. Minor LB, Schessel DA, Carey JP (2004) Meniere's disease. Curr Opin Neurol 17(1):9–16

7. Ohki M, Matsuzaki M, Sugasawa K, Murofushi T (2002) Vestibular evoked myogenic potentials in ipsila delayed endolymphatic hydrops. J Otorhinolaryngol Relat Spec 64(6):424–428

8. Sando I, Orita Y, Hirsch BE (2002) Pathology and pathophysiology of Meniere's disease. Otolaryngol Clin North Am 35(3):517–528

Benign Positional Vertigo

9

Core Messages

> BPPV is the most common peripheral vestibular disorder.

> The pathophysiology of BPPV has favoured either canalolithasis (free floating particles) or cupuloithiasis (particulate debris attached to the cupula).

> Atypical BPPV requires exclusion of posterior fossa pathology.

> Habituation exercises (Brandt-Daroff), physical therapy manoeurves (Eply and particle repositioning procedures) and semicircular canal occlusion surgery represent available treatments.

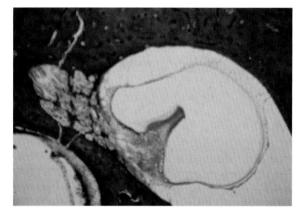

Fig. 9.1 Ampulla of the posterior semicircular canal

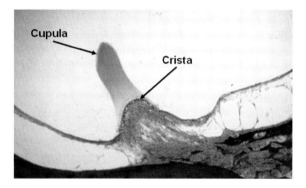

Fig. 9.2 Section demonstrating the normal ampulla of the posterior semicircular canal

Benign paroxysmal positional vertigo (BPPV) is the most common cause of vertigo arising from peripheral vestibular dysfunction. Its prevalence increases with age but is often underestimated in older adults [5].

While numerous theories have been postulated for its occurrence, the most widely accepted theory for BPPV (and related disorders) involves the deposition of calcium carbonate crystals (from degenerated otoliths) from the utricular macula that float freely in the endolymph of the semicircular canals (so-called canalothiasis). The free-floating particles usually enter into the posterior semicircular canal circulation which is the most gravity-dependent canal or more rarely, the horizontal or superior canals (Figs. 9.1 and 9.2).

The free-floating debris is felt to be hyperdense relative to the endolymph. With a change of the head position primarily in the plane of the posterior semicircular canal (i.e., looking up, bending over, rolling over in bed, etc.), gravitational forces cause the crystals to migrate inside the canal. This in turn induces a transitory endolymph drag with a consequent cupullar deflection, which will produce an attack of short-lived vertigo (typically lasting for seconds) and nystagmus.

M. M. Zarandy and J. Rutka, *Diseases of the Inner Ear*
DOI: 10.1007/978-3-642-05058-9_9, © Springer-Verlag Berlin Heidelberg 2010

Nystagmus patterns in BPPV from canalolithiasis have a characteristic latency of onset, direction (geotropic rotatory), appear transitory, reverse with return to the original position (ageotropic reversal), and are fatigable with repetitive provocation.

The term cupulolithiasis is applied when particulate debris usually attaches to the cupula of the posterior semicircular canal, rendering it sensitive to positional change. Canalolithiasis is said to occur when particular debris floats freely within the semicircular canal [4]. On clinical grounds, the persistence of nystgamus with positional change is more likely to reflect the phenomenon of cupulolithiasis from continued deflection of the cupula (Figs. 9.3–9.9).

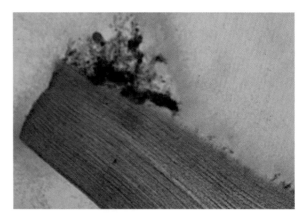

Fig. 9.5 Cupulolithiasis

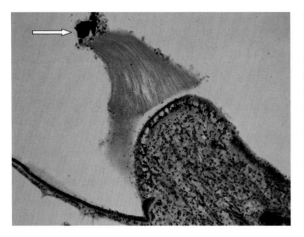

Fig. 9.3 Cupulolithiasis. Note the basophilic staining debris on the cupulla. See *arrow*

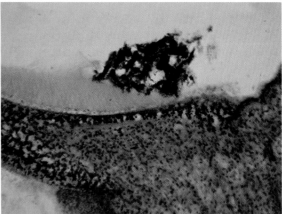

Fig. 9.6 Basophilic staining debris on the utricular macula

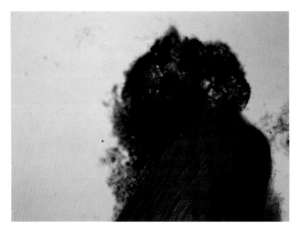

Fig. 9.4 Cupulolithiasis. Higher magnification

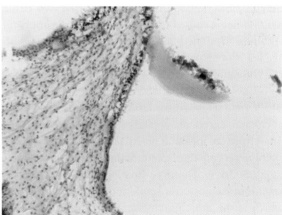

Fig. 9.7 Cupulolithiasis. Particulate debris attached to the cupulla renders it gravity-sensitive resulting from a provocative head movement

Fig. 9.8 Canalolithiasis. Free floating particles noted within the opened posterior semicircular canal of a patient undergoing a non-ampullary posterior semicircular canal occlusion surgery for intractable BPPV. Courtesy of Dr Lorne Parnes. See *arrows*

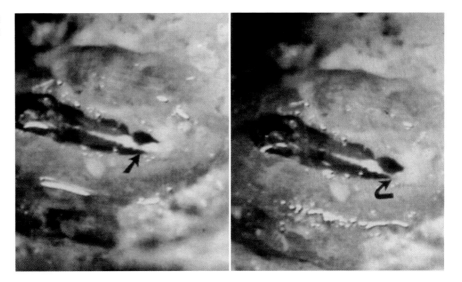

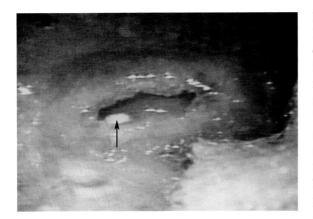

Fig. 9.9 Canalolithiasis. See *arrow.* Courtesy of Dr Lorne Parnes

A diagnosis for posterior canal BPPV from canalolithaisis is based on the clinical findings of a transient, up-beating (or geotropic) torsional nystagmus with the upper poles of the eyes beating toward the undermost ear in Dix-Hallpike test. The differential diagnosis of the positional vertigo and nystagmus can be challenging at times especially when atypical features are present [2]. A diagnosis for horizontal canal BPPV due to canalolithiasis is made when a direction-changing lateral nystagmus beating in the horizontal (toward the lower ear) direction is identified when the head is in lateral position, while the patient is supine. The nystagmus is less transitory, usually lasts longer than in the posterior canal BPV, and takes longer to fatigue. To confuse matters, another variant of the horizontal canal cupulolithiasis has been described. In this variant, the nystagmus changes direction, is permanent, has no latency, is not fatigable, and beats in the apo-geotropic (toward the upper ear) direction when the patient is lying down. These features of the nystagmus are also seen in the posterior fossa lesions and pathology making it difficult at times to differentiate the horizontal canal involvement from central etiologies [1, 3].

Historically, Brandt-Daroff exercises have been recommended for patients with suspected cupulolithiasis. If canalolithiasis is suspected, then the treatment usually requires "liberatory" or "particle repositioning" maneuvers. Both the physical therapies aim to move the displaced otoconia out of the semicircular canal circulation to another location within the vestibular labyrinth. Surgical treatments such as the occlusion of the posterior semicircular canal are sometimes required when BPPV proves recalcitrant to physical and medical therapies (Figs. 9.10–9.14).

Fig. 9.10 Brandt-Daroff exercises for BPPV arising from cupulolithiasis

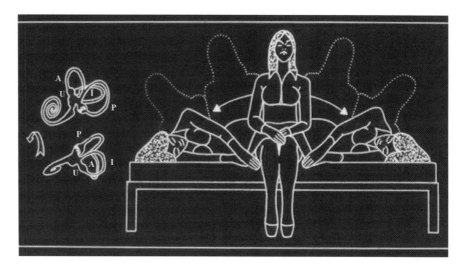

Fig. 9.11 Particle repositioning maneuver for canalolithiasis involving the right posterior semicircular canal **a**. upright position with particulate debris (canalolithiasis) in posterior semicircular canal (PSCC), **b**. right Dix-Hallpikes manouvre with movement of debris in PSCC, **c**. left head rotation with continued movement of particulate debris, **d**. return of particulate debris into vestibule in head down position

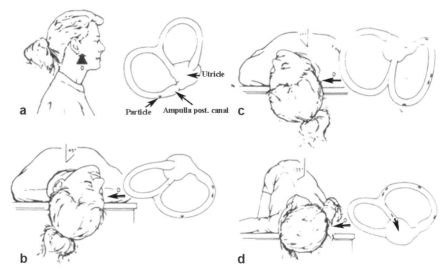

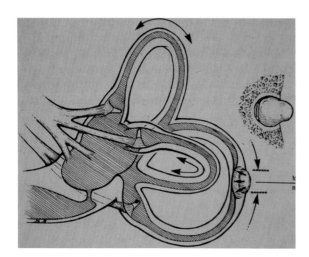

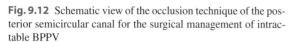

Fig. 9.12 Schematic view of the occlusion technique of the posterior semicircular canal for the surgical management of intractable BPPV

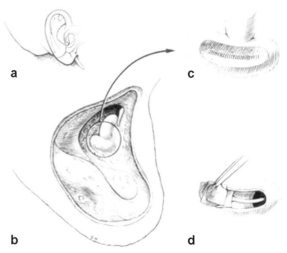

Fig. 9.13 Schematic representation of the posterior semicircular canal occlusion **a**. Right mastoidectomy approach, **b**. cortical mastoidectomy with identification of PSCC, **c**. blue line with fenestration into PSCC, **d**. occlusion of PSCC with autogenous periosteum

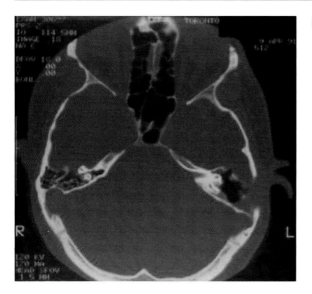

Fig. 9.14 Axial CT demonstrating an occluded left posterior semicircular canal post mastoidectomy approach

References

1. Bisdorff AR, Debatisse D (2001) Localizing signs in positional vertigo due to lateral canal cupulolithiasis. Neurology 57(6):1085–1088
2. Del Rio M, Arriaga MA (2004) Benign positional vertigo: prognostic factors. Otolaryngol Head Neck Surg 130(4): 426–429
3. Haynes DS, Resser JR, Labadie RF, Girasole CR, Kovach BT, Scheker LE, Walker DC (2002) Treatment of benign positional vertigo using the semont maneuver: efficacy in patients presenting without nystagmus. Laryngoscope 112(5):796–801
4. Parnes LS, McClure JA (1992) Free floating endolymph particles: a new operative finding during posterior semicircular canal occlusion. Laryngoscope 102:988–992
5. Salvinelli F, Trivelli M, Casale M, Firrisi L, Di Peco V, D'Ascanio L, Greco F, Miele A, Petitti T, Bernabei R (2004) Treatment of benign positional vertigo in the elderly: a randomized trial. Laryngoscope 114(5):827–831

Meningioma

Core Messages

> Meningiomas are the 2nd most common benign CP angle tumor after vestibular schwannomas.

> Both endogenous (gene mutations) and exogenous (ionizing radiation, hormones) factors have been implicated in their development.

> Meningiomas can usually be differentiated on CT/MRI findings from vestibular schwannomas.

> The differential diagnosis for a reddened middle ear mass includes a meningioma.

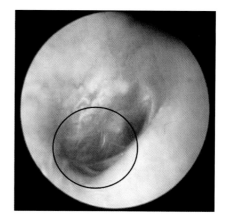

Fig. 10.1 Skull base (inferior) meningioma with extension into the middle ear. Differential diagnosis would include a glomus tumor or dehiscent internal carotid artery. See *circle*

Meningiomas are benign tumors composed of neoplastic meningothelial (arachnoidal cap) cells. They constitute approximately 20% of all primary intracranial tumors with an approximate annual incidence of 6 per 100,000 population. After acoustic tumors, meningiomas are the second most common cerebellopontine (CP) angle tumor accounting for approximately 10–15% of the lesions in this area. The peak incidence is between the sixth and seventh decades of life. They are more frequent in women than in men with a 2:1 ratio. The majority of meningiomas are attached to the dura matter and arise within the intracranial cavity, the spinal canal, or rarely, the orbit. They can extend extracranially throughout the skull base. Some meningiomas may arise primarily as intraosseous tumors. Clinical symptoms depend on the location of the tumor [2] (Figs. 10.1 and 10.2).

Several endogenous and exogenous factors that predispose to meningioma development have been identified.

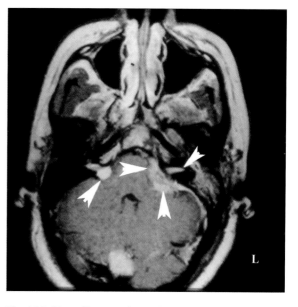

Fig. 10.2 Neurofibromatosis type 2. Left posterior fossa meningioma (multiple *arrows*) in a patient with right vestibular schwannoma (solitary *arrow*). Note the dural tail along the left temporal bone

M. M. Zarandy and J. Rutka, *Diseases of the Inner Ear*
DOI: 10.1007/978-3-642-05058-9_10, © Springer-Verlag Berlin Heidelberg 2010

The majority of patients with neurofibromatosis type 2 (NF2) develop meningiomas. Mutations in the *NF2* tumor suppressor gene located in the chromosomal region 22q12.2 represent the most frequent gene alteration in meningiomas. In addition, families with an increased susceptibility to meningiomas but without NF2 have been reported [3].

Ionizing radiation and sex hormones are reported as exogenous factors.

These lesions can be divided into six categories according to their site, namely: lateral, midpetrosal, internal auditory meatal, petroclival, Meckel's area, and inferior. Histologically, meningiomas can be divided into three main classes: meningotheliomatous, fibroblastic, and malignant.

On CT, meningiomas appear as well-demarcated lesions related to the petrous bone, usually with a broad base against the bone. They are isodense to hyperdense compared to the adjacent brain. Intratumor calcification is a common finding. Enhancement is usually strong and homogeneous. Cystic lesions are uncommon. Brain compression may be present to varying degrees depending on the tumor size. As most tumors are slow growing, they often reach a considerable size before causing clinical symptoms (Figs. 10.3 and 10.4).

On MRI, meningiomas may be isointense to the brain on T1-weighted images. On T2-weighted images, they can be isointense, hypointense, or even hyperintense. Cystic components are present and may be located in the center or the periphery of the tumor. A cerebrospinal fluid (CSF) cleft may separate the lesion from the adjacent brain. Contrast enhancement in meningiomas is usually obvious and homogeneous.

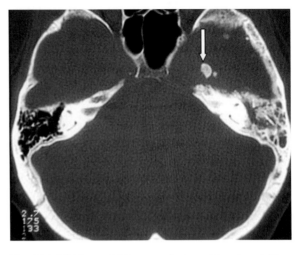

Fig. 10.4 Middle cranial fossa meningioma. Note the calcifications (see *arrow*)

The typical feature of meningiomas includes the dural tail enhancement that may extend for a variable distance from the lesion (Figs. 10.5 and 10.6).

The clinical presentation of a CP-angle meningioma is similar to an acoustic tumor. Based on clinical and otological grounds, differentiation of these two entities is often impossible. Hearing loss, however, is generally more profound with a schwannoma, whereas symptoms due to trigeminal nerve compression are more common with meningiomas [4].

The differential diagnosis for a meningioma when it extends into the middle ear includes a paraganglioma (glomus tumor), schwannoma, carcinoma, and middle-ear adenoma (Figs. 10.7 and 10.8).

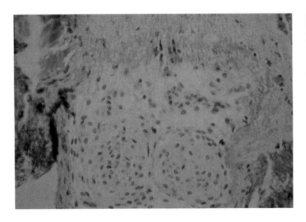

Fig. 10.3 Meningiotheliomatous pattern in meningioma. Note the distinct whorls of the tumor cells

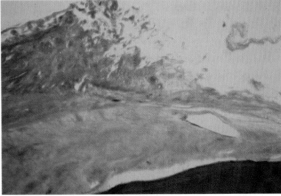

Fig. 10.5 Middle cranial fossa meningioma. Note the apparent dural thickening

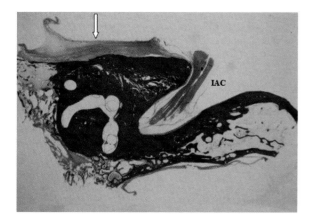

Fig. 10.6 Posterior cranial fossa meningioma with extension towards the internal auditory canal (see *arrow*). *IAC* internal auditory canal

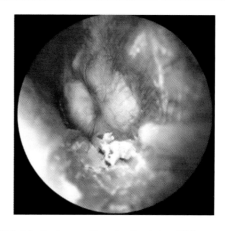

Fig. 10.8 Meningioma with extension into middle ear causing erosion of the tympanic bone inferiorly

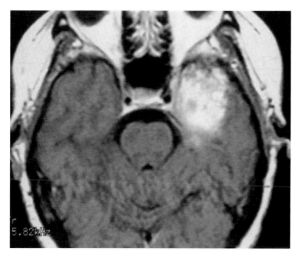

Fig. 10.7 Middle cranial fossa meningioma (an MRI image)

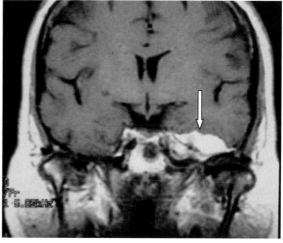

Fig. 10.9 Middle cranial fossa meningioma on contrast-enhanced MRI (see *arrow*)

In contrast, the differentiation of a meningioma from a schwannoma based on their radiological appearances is possible. In general, meningiomas rarely expand to the internal auditory canal (IAC), usually have a broad base along the petrous bone (dural tail), and have strong homogeneous contrast enhancement. They are usually hyperdense on noncontrast CT. Calcification and extension to Meckle's cave or the jugular foramen are more commonly seen with meningiomas [5].

In general, schwannomas are hypodense on noncontrast CT, enhance less homogeneously, and typically cause a widening of the IAC. Calcification is rare in schwannomas (Fig. 10.9).

Unless symptoms dictate, most meningiomas are monitored conservatively. When active intervention is required, total surgical excision (if possible) is usually recommended. Within the posterior fossa and cerebellopontine angle, a retrosigmoid (suboccipital) is generally favored over a translabyrinthine approach.

Conventional radiotherapy and gamma-knife radiosurgery may be used as adjuvant therapeutic modalities under certain conditions [1, 4].

References

1. Altinors N, Caner H, Bavbek M, Erdogan B, Atalay B, Calisaneller T, Cekinmez M (2004) Problems in the management of intracranial meningiomas. J Invest Surg 17(5):283–289

2. Lamszus K (2004) Meningioma pathology, genetics, and biology. J Neuropathol Exp Neurol 63(4):275–286

3. Lin CC, Kenyon L, Hyslop T, Hammond E, Andrews DW, Curran WJ Jr, Dicker AP (2003) Cyclooxygenase-2 (COX-2) expression in human meningioma as a function of tumor grade. Am J Clin Oncol 26(4):S98–S102

4. Thompson LD, Bouffard JP, Sandberg GD, Mena H (2003) Primary ear and temporal bone meningiomas: a clinico-pathologic study of 36 cases with a review of the literature. Mod Pathol 16(3):236–245

5. Zamani AA (2000) Cerebellopontine angle tumors: role of magnetic resonance imaging. Top Magn Reson Imaging 11(2):98–107

Vestibular Schwannoma

Core Messages

> Vestibular schwannomas (acoustic neuromas) are the most common benign CP angle tumor.

> Most unilateral VS's arise sporadically; bilateral VS's implies neurofibromatosis type II (NF-II) arising from genetic mutations on chromosone 22.

> Wishart and Gardner NF-II phenotypes have significantly different clinical outcomes.

> Gadolinium enhanced MRI scanning remains "the gold standard" for diagnosis.

> Treatment options include conservative management ("wait and scan"), microsurgical removal or focussed stereotactic radiation. All have specific benefits and risks.

Vestibular schwannomas account for 80% of all cerebellopontine (CP) angle tumors. The peak incidence of presentation is between the fourth and sixth decades of life. There is no known sexual predilection. Their etiology remains unknown. Most unilateral vestibular schwannomas arise sporadically. Bilateral presentation usually implies the autosomal dominant condition of neurofibromatosis II (NF II) with gene abnormalities on chromosome 22 [5].

Pathologically, vestibular schwannomas are usually round or semi-oval encapsulated lesions that arise from the Schwann cells at the neurolemmal–neuroglial junction (where the peripheral myelin meets the CNS myelin) of the vestibular nerve. The junction is usually found in the internal auditory canal (IAC) and explains why most vestibular schwannomas arise there initially.

While benign, vestibular schwannomas tend to grow slowly. With progressive growth, they can extend into the CP angle causing compression of the brainstem and the surrounding cranial nerves [2] (Figs. 11.1–11.4).

Light microscopy of vestibular schwannomas demonstrates two different histopathologic patterns: Antoni A and Antoni B.

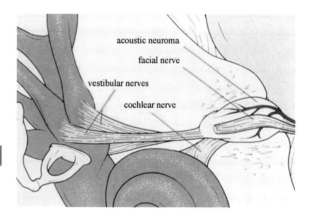

Fig. 11.1 Intracanalicular vestibular schwannoma. Schematic diagram

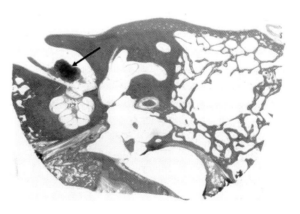

Fig. 11.2 Intracanalicular vestibular schwannoma. See *arrow*

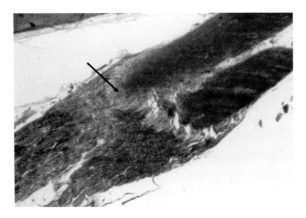

Fig. 11.3 Neurolemma–neuroglia junction. See *arrow*

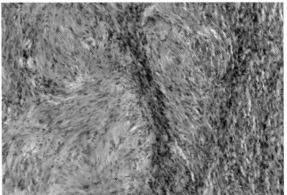

Fig. 11.5 Vestibular schwannoma demonstrating Antoni A configuration. Note the tightly packed cells with a whirling and pallisading appearance

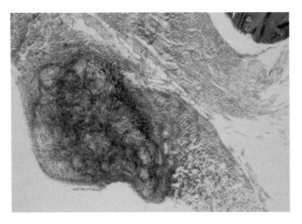

Fig. 11.4 Vestibular schwannoma arising from neurolemma–neuroglia junction in the internal auditory canal

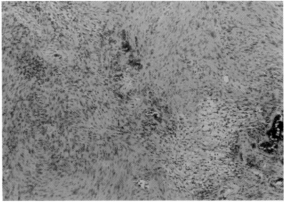

Fig. 11.6 Vestibular schwannoma demonstrating Antoni B configuration. Note the loosely packed and vacuolated cells which are thought to represent a degenerative process

Antoni A configurations demonstrate schwann cells that are densely packed in a whirling or pallisading fashion. They typically have an elongated bipolar appearance with club-shaped nuclei. Antoni B configurations consist of a loose aggregate of stellar cells with abundant lipid. Cystic degeneration is frequently seen, especially in larger tumors. Other pathologic degenerative changes include thickened and hyalinized vessels, xanthomatous cells, and hemosiderin-loaded macrophages. Verocay bodies are described when pallisading cells line up against each other in a "rail-road track" appearance. It is not unusual to see both Antoni A and B configurations in the same tumor [2] (Figs. 11.5 and 11.6).

Patients with vestibular schwannomas usually present with a progressive unilateral sensorineural hearing loss (sudden hearing loss is said to occur in approximately 1–2% of patients with a vestibular schwannoma).

As the tumor grows into the CP angle, other presenting symptoms may include facial numbness, dysphagia/hoarseness (from lower cranial nerve involvement), and headaches (from obstructive or communicating hydrocephalus), particularly when the tumor is greater than 3 cm in size. Despite the close involvement of the tumor with the facial nerve, facial nerve paralysis is a relatively late finding. Vertigo is also relatively uncommon although the patients not infrequently complain of a generalized unsteadiness (Figs. 11.7–11.10).

Clinical suspicion of a vestibular schwannoma warrants an imaging investigation for confirmation or exclusion. Both computerized tomography (CT) and magnetic resonance imaging (MRI) can be employed. MRI is especially sensitive for soft tissue differentiation and is ideally suited for the identification of extra-axial lesions within the IAC and CP angle. CT

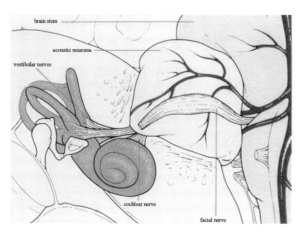

Fig. 11.7 Schematic diagram of a large vestibular schwannoma causing brainstem compression

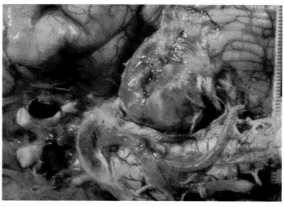

Fig. 11.9 Large left vestibular schwannoma causing brainstem and cerebellar compression. Note the effects of the tumor on the surrounding cranial nerves and the vertebrobasilar system

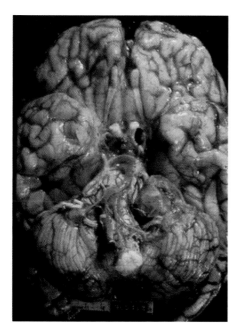

Fig. 11.8 Large left vestibular schwannoma causing brainstem and cerebellar compression

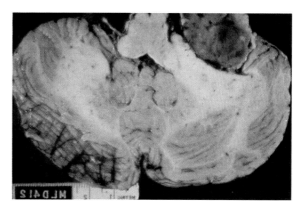

Fig. 11.10 Large left vestibular schwannoma. Cerebellum is compressed and the fourth ventricle is shifted to the right of the midline

may be more likely to demonstrate a bony change such as an enlarged IAC.

MRI techniques and resolution capabilities have dramatically improved over the past several years. This in turn has led to a trend for the earlier detection, precise localization, and size evaluation of these tumors. Vestibular schwannomas appear isointense to hypointense to the brain on T1-weighted images (T1-WI). They are hyperintense and may be inhomogeneous on T2-weighted images (T2-WI). Inhomogeneity may reflect cystic degeneration, hemorrhage, or the intralesional vascularity of the tumor. According to T2-WI and post-gadolinium T1-WI, the three different MRI appearances of the tumoral tissue are frequently described as homogeneous, heterogeneous, or cystic [1–3, 7].

While the most common cause for gadolinium contrast enhancement within the IAC is a vestibular schwannoma, this is by no means pathognomonic (Figs. 11.11–11.13).

On CT, vestibular schwannomas appear either isodense or hypodense to the adjacent brain. The porus acusticus is often widened. Enhancement of these lesions is fairly intense and usually homogeneous, although large lesions may show an inhomogeneous enhancement. Calcification is extremely rare and would be more likely present in a meningioma (Figs. 11.14 and 11.15).

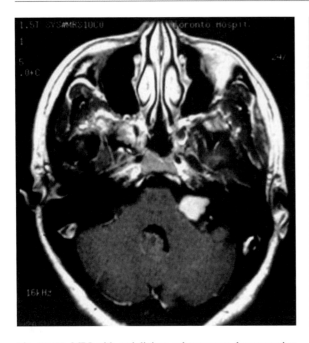

Fig. 11.11 MRI with gadolinium enhancement demonstrating vestibular schwannoma

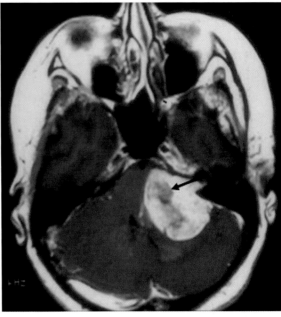

Fig. 11.13 Large vestibular schwannoma in cerebellopontine angle. Central portion of the tumor reveals areas of necrosis. See *arrow*

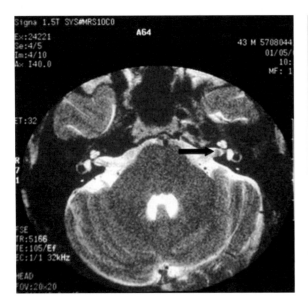

Fig. 11.12 MRI demonstrating small intracanalicular vestibular schwannoma. See *arrow*

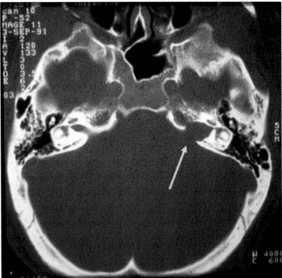

Fig. 11.14 Enlarged internal auditory canal in a patient with a vestibular schwannoma. See *arrow*

Management options in the treatment of an individual with a solitary vestibular schwannoma include a trial of conservative management ("wait and scan"), stereotactic radiosurgery, or microsurgical removal. All these can be considered as valid options depending on the age of the patient, the size of the tumor, presence of serviceable hearing, comorbid health issues, and the patient's expectations [6].

When microsurgical removal is indicated, total tumor removal with minimal morbidity is the main aim in treatment. Continued advances in microsurgical techniques have meant that the removal of even a giant tumor (defined as greater than 4 cm) can be successfully achieved with minimal mortality. The patient's hearing, the tumor location, and its size influence the choice of the microsurgical approach. In general terms, serviceable

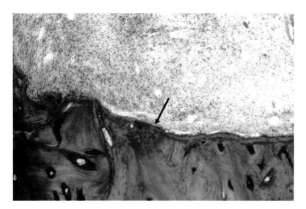

Fig. 11.15 Vestibular schwannoma at the interface with the bone of the internal auditory canal (IAC). It is unlikely that the pressure effects from the tumor growth cause an expansion of the IAC. See *arrow*

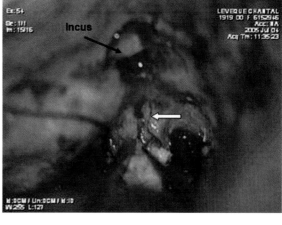

Fig. 11.17 Translabyrithine approach demonstrating the VII nerve in the labyrinthine segment (see *arrow*)

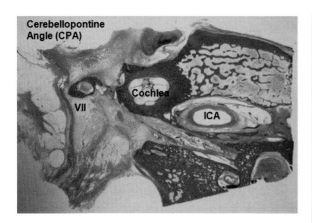

Fig. 11.16 Cadaveric specimen. Translabyrithine approach for the removal of a vestibular schwannoma demonstrating that the labyrinth has been removed with the anatomical preservation of the facial nerve in its vertical segment. *ICA* internal carotid artery; *VII* facial nerve

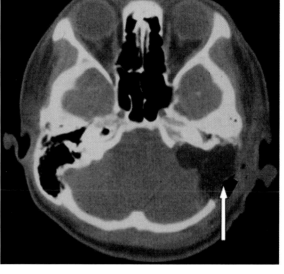

Fig. 11.18 Postoperative translabyrinthine resection for an acoustic neuroma. Abdominal fat has been placed into the mastoid craniectomy postoperatively. See *arrow*

hearing has a better chance of being preserved in an affected ear when the tumor is small and detected early. Anatomical preservation of the facial nerve is possible in up to 95% of patients in tumors less than 2 cm. Procedures in the microsurgical armamentarium for tumor removal include retrosigmoid (suboccipital), translabyrinthine, and middle-fossa approaches. The indication for a specific microsurgical approach will depend on the size of the tumor, skill of the surgical team, the anatomy of the temporal bone, and whether hearing preservation is a realistic goal [4] (Figs. 11.16–11.19).

In NF II, the prevailing trend is to conservatively manage the tumors and to only intervene when progressive tumor growth affects other cranial nerves or causes significant cerebellar/brainstem compression. Radiation is usually avoided as there have been reported instances of malignant transformation following radiotherapy. While genetic testing in NF II has demonstrated abnormalities on chromosome 22, on clinical grounds, there are two major presenting phenotypes, namely the Gardner and Wishart variants. The Gardner variant of NF II has a favorable prognosis for longevity, and the involved individuals tend to present with bilateral vestibular schwannomas later in life. In the Wishart variant, younger patients present with rapidly growing vestibular schwannomas, typically associated with multiple intracranial and extracranial nerve tumors (Figs. 11.20–11.24).

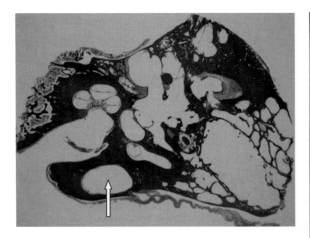

Fig. 11.19 High jugular bulb (see *arrow*) would pose a relative contraindication to the translabyrithine removal of a vestibular schwannoma. *IAC* internal auditory canal; *VII* facial nerve

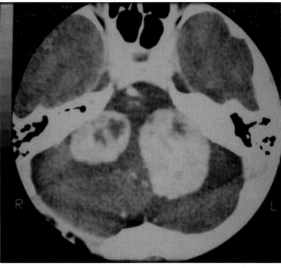

Fig. 11.20 Neurofibromatosis (NF II) with bilateral acoustic neuromas (Wishart's variant)

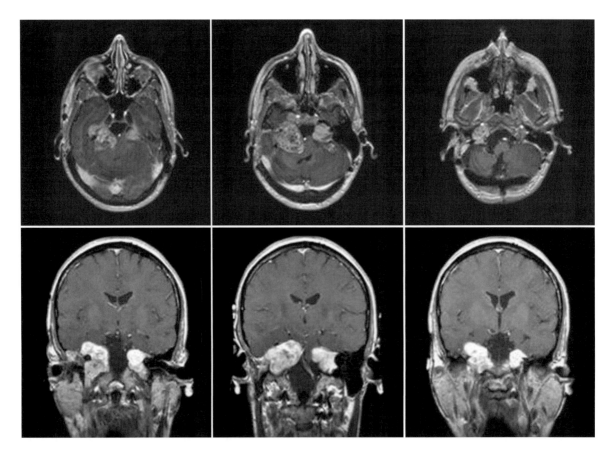

Fig. 11.21 Neurofibromatosis (NF II) with bilateral acoustic neuromas. Patient also demonstrating bilateral trigeminal schwannomas in addition (Wishart's variant)

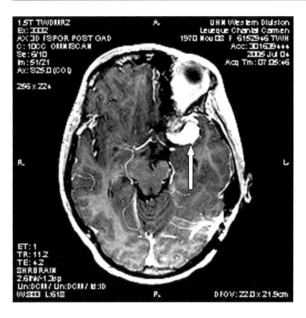

Fig. 11.22 Tumor of the orbit apex in a patient with NF II (see *arrow*)

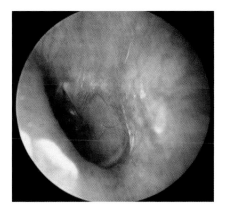

Fig. 11.23 Unusual otoscopic finding of an acoustic neuroma in the left middle ear in a patient with NF II. Tumor had extended from the vestibule into the middle ear

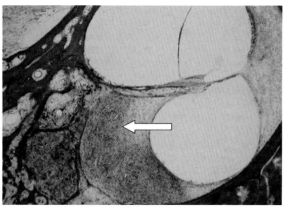

Fig. 11.24 Intracochlear schwannoma in a patient with NF II (see *arrow*)

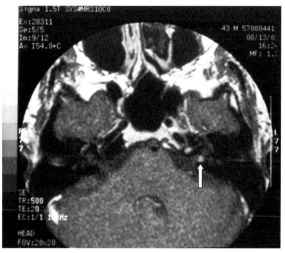

Fig. 11.25 Conservative management of a left intracanalicular vestibular schwannoma in a patient observed for 3 years. No significant growth in tumor was identified on serial MRI imaging (see *arrow*)

Some recent studies have emphasized the role of conservative management in selected cases of vestibular schwannomas (1). This is on the basis that most tumors grow slowly, typically within the order of 1–2 mm/year within the CP angle and the quality of life studies which usually demonstrate that patients feel best if nothing active is required. Should this treatment option be embarked upon, it is mandatory that repeat imaging studies are carried out for the patient. Unless contraindicated, MRI is the modality of choice for follow-up in patients with vestibular schwannomas (Fig. 11.25).

Focused stereotactic radiosurgery (FSR) is yet another option for the patient to consider. In FSR, the goal is to biologically sterilize the tumor such that it does not grow (although it will always be present). Radiosurgery treatment options include Gamma-knife (where the patient receives a single highly concentrated focused dose of radiation to their tumor) vs. LINAC (where multiple fractionations of the lower dose radiation is received over a 4–6 week timeframe) radiosurgery. In conclusion, when tumors are less than 3 cm in size, radiation is approximately 85–90% successful in stopping a tumor from growing.

References

1. Daniels RL, Swallow C, Shelton C, Davidson HC, Krejci CS, Harnsberger HR (2000) Causes of unilateral sensorineural hearing loss screened by high-resolution fast spin echo magnetic resonance imaging: review of 1,070 consecutive cases. Am J Otol 21(2):173–180
2. Gomez-Brouchet A, Delisle MB, Cognard C, Bonafe A, Charlet JP, Deguine O, Fraysse B (2001) Vestibular schwannomas: correlations between magnetic resonance imaging and histopathologic appearance. Otol Neurotol 22(1):79–86
3. Hasegawa T, Kida Y, Kobayashi T, Yoshimoto M, Mori Y, Yoshida J (2005) Long-term outcomes in patients with vestibular schwannomas treated using gamma knife surgery: 10-year follow up. J Neurosurg 102(1):10–16
4. Mamikoglu B, Wiet RJ, Esquivel CR (2002) Translabyrinthine approach for the management of large and giant vestibular schwannomas. Otol Neurotol 23(2):224–227
5. Mohyuddin A, Vokurka EA, Evans DG, Ramsden RT, Jackson A (2003) Is clinical growth index a reliable predictor of tumour growth in vestibular schwannomas? Otolaryngol Allied Sci 28(2):85–90
6. Raut VV, Walsh RM, Bath AP, Bance ML, Guha A, Tator CH, Rutka JA (2004) Conservative management of vestibular schwannomas – second review of a prospective longitudinal study. Clin Otolaryngol Allied Sci 29(5):505–514
7. Zamani AA (2000) Cerebellopontine angle tumors: role of magnetic resonance imaging. Top Magn Reson Imaging 11(2):98–107

Other Cranial Nerve Schwannomas and Paragangliomas

12

Core Messages

> Recurrent episodes of unilateral "Bell's palsy" requires exclusion of a facial nerve schwannoma.

> Tympanojugular paragangiomas (glomus tumors) classically present with a pulsatile tinnitus and a red middle ear mass.

> Molecular research has identified 4 hereditary paraganglioma syndromes that arise from mutations in succinate dehydrogenase (SDH) genes.

> Treatment options (conservative management, microsurgical removal or radiation) depend on the location, extent of disease involvement and patient factors.

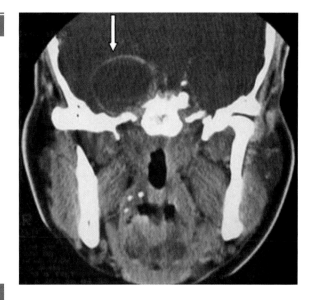

Fig. 12.1 Trigeminal nerve schwannoma (*arrow*)

Schwannomas may affect the temporal bone and inner ear when they arise on cranial nerves V, VII. IX, X, XI, and XII. Vestibular schwannomas, however, still remain the most common tumor of schwann cell origin [6].

Trigeminal schwannomas initially present with pain and numbness in trigeminal distribution. Patients with a facial schwannoma may present with recurrent episodes of "Bell's" palsy or a progressive conductive hearing loss in addition to a mass in the posterior superior quadrant of the tympanic membrane. Patients with lower cranial nerve (IX–XII) schwannomas not infrequently present with findings suggestive of a glomus jugular tumor. Their presenting symptoms are typically those of vocal change, hoarseness, and/or dysphagia [1, 2] (Figs. 12.1–12.13).

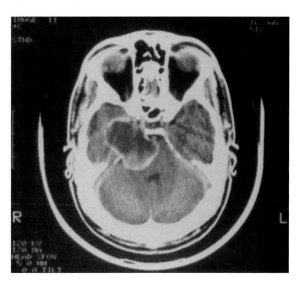

Fig. 12.2 Trigeminal neuroma straddling petrous apex. Same patient as in Fig. 12.1

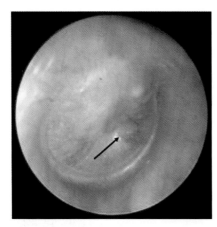

Fig. 12.3 Facial nerve schwannoma involving the horizontal segment of the facial nerve, presenting as a mass in the posterior superior quadrant of the tympanic membrane. See *arrow*

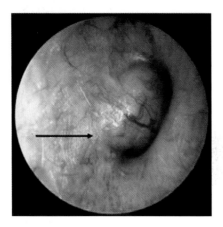

Fig. 12.4 Facial nerve (VII) schwannoma (2.5 years after diagnosis). See *arrow*

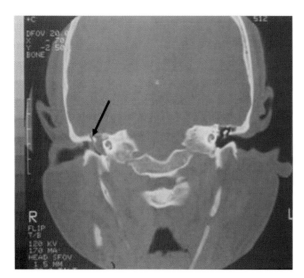

Fig. 12.5 Facial nerve (VII) schwannoma (2.5 years after diagnosis) Same patient as in Fig. 12.3. See *arrow*

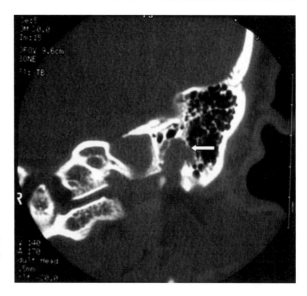

Fig. 12.6 Facial nerve (VII) schwannoma involving the vertical segment of the facial nerve on the coronal CT scan. See *arrow*

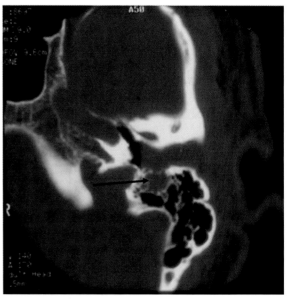

Fig. 12.7 Axial CT scan of the temporal bone demonstrating the expanded VII nerve canal secondary to facial nerve schwannoma. Same patient as in Fig. 12.6. See *arrow*

Paragangliomas are benign, yet locally erosive tumors that arise from chemoreceptive tissue of the parasympathetic nervous system. They are commonly found along the course of Jacobson's plexus in the middle ear, the dome of the jugular bulb, and along the course of the vagus nerve in the neck down to the arch of the aorta. Their location and origin primarily

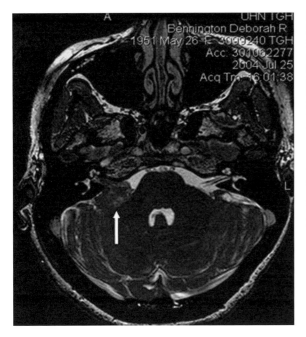

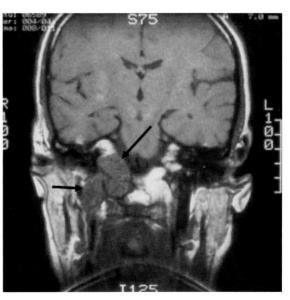

Fig. 12.10 Right hypoglossal schwannoma demonstrating intracranial and extracranial tumor extension. Same patient as in Fig. 12.9. See *arrows*

Fig. 12.8 Vestibular schwannoma (acoustic neuroma). The tumor is centered and typically begins in the internal auditory canal extending into the cerebellopontine angle. See *arrow*

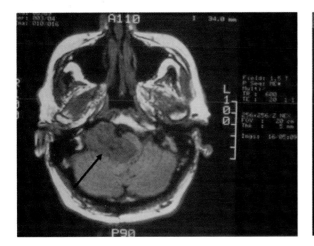

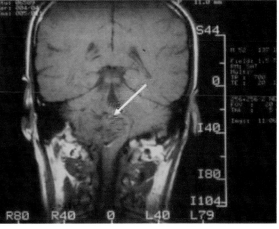

Fig. 12.9 Axial MRI scan demonstrating the right hypoglossal schwannoma causing significant brainstem compression. See *arrow*

Fig. 12.11 Coronal MRI demonstrating significant cerebellar compression. Same patient as in Fig. 12.9. See *arrow*

determine their classification. The term glomus tumor is used interchangeably.

A glomus tympanicum tumor represents a small localized paraganglioma confined to the middle ear space. Clinically, it may present as an incidental well-circumscribed red mass behind an intact tympanic membrane. On other occasions, it may cause a conductive hearing loss and be associated with a roaring pulsatile tinnitus [2, 5].

A glomus jugulare tumor, conversely, is more likely to be larger, arising within the adventitia of the jugular bulb. This tumor frequently involves the lower cranial nerves (IX–XI) resulting in numerous cranial nerve palsies. Its appearance in the middle ear is usually a late occurrence after it has broken through the hypotympanic floor. A pulsatile bruit is typically heard over the temporal bone in affected individuals. Presentation of the tumor as a pulsatile, red aural "polyp" should be

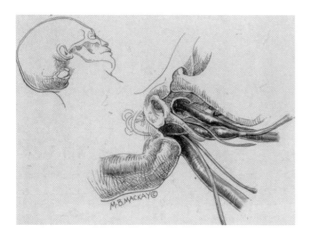

Fig. 12.12 Schematic diagram of the normal neural and vascular skull base lateral skull base anatomy

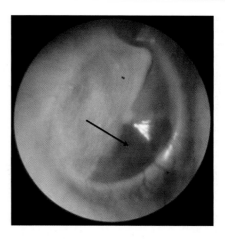

Fig. 12.14 Glomus tympanicum tumor. See *arrow*

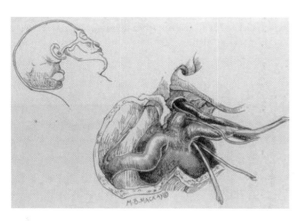

Fig. 12.13 Schematic diagram of the right hypoglossal schwannoma demonstrating its intracranial and extracranial involvement. Same patient as in Fig. 12.9

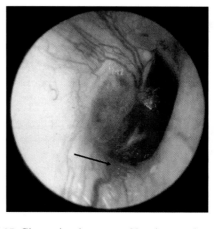

Fig. 12.15 Glomus jugulare tumor. Note increased vascularity along the floor of the ear canal. See *arrow*

approached with care as biopsy is often associated with profuse bleeding [3, 5] (Figs. 12.14–12.19).

Glomus vagale tumors arise from the vascular tissues that accompany the vagus nerve in the neck. With upward extension, they may erode into the middle ear where they are indistinguishable from a glomus jugulare. Findings of a unilateral vocal cord paralysis remain their most common presentation. The diagnosis is usually made on their location from imaging studies (Figs. 12.20 and 12.21).

Histologically, a glomus tumor consists of a dense network of thin-walled sinusoidal capillaries that surround glomerular or alveolar-like nests of tumor cells.

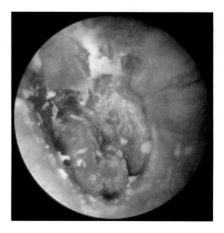

Fig. 12.16 Glomus jugulare tumor demonstrating the erosion of the tumor into the ear canal presenting as a pusatile, highly vascular aural polyp

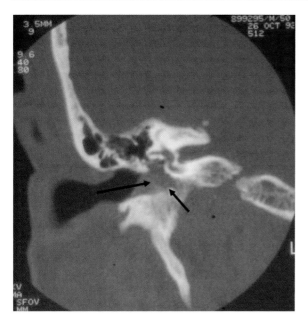

Fig. 12.17 Glomus jugulare. Coronal CT scan demonstrating a soft tissue mass in the right middle ear with bony change in the tympanic bone inferiorly. See *arrows*

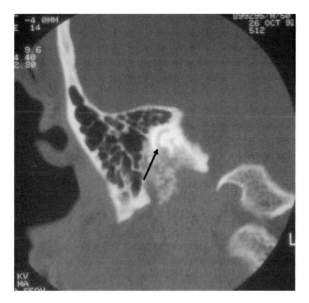

Fig. 12.18 Glomus jugulare. Coronal CT scan demonstrating the erosion of the tumor into the posterior semicircular canal and skull base. Same patient as in Fig. 12.17. See *arrow*

The tumor cells have a clear or eosinophilic cytoplasm. Under electron microscopy, one can see numerous electron dense, round neurosecretory granules within the cytoplasm. Molecular research has described 4 hereditary paraganglioma syndromes (PGL 1-4) to

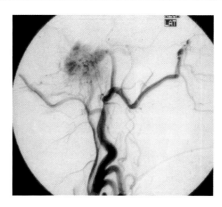

Fig. 12.19 Glomus jugulare. Selective cerebral angiogram demonstrating tumor blush primarily arising from the ascending pharyngeal and temporal arteries. Same patient as in Fig. 12.17

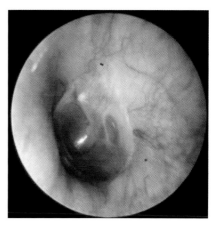

Fig. 12.20 Glomus vagale. Patient presented with a pulsatile tinnitus and a unilateral vocal cord paralysis

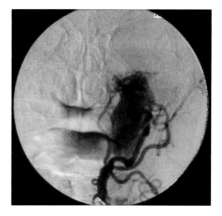

Fig. 12.21 Glomus vagale. Angiogram demonstrates an intense vascularity of the tumor in the upper neck with extension into the middle ear

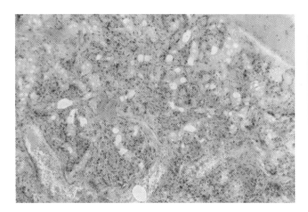

Fig. 12.22 Histology of a glomus tumor demonstrating the numerous thin-walled sinusoidal capillaries

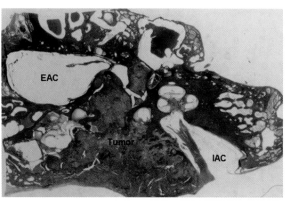

Fig. 12.23 Glomus tumor extending and eroding into the mastoid, internal auditory canal (IAC), and external auditory canal (EAC)

date arising from mutations in succinate dehydrogenase (SDH) genes. SDH genes act as tumor suppressors. When mutated they appear to cause an overexpression of hypoxia-inducible genes which results in proliferation of paraganglioma tissue. Approximately 30% of sporadic head and neck paragangiomas have germ line mutations (Fig. 12.22) [1].

The treatment of a glomus tumor will largely depend on its location, the extent of the disease, and patient factors (i.e., age, comorbid health related issues, etc.). Glomus tympanicum tumors are often observed but can usually be removed quite safely when necessary via an extended tympanotomy approach. For larger tumors of the glomus jugulare or vagale type, preoperative embolization is often recommended to decrease tumor vascularity intraoperatively. Surgical removal requires an extensive exposure of the temporal bone with neck exploration to gain control of the feeding blood vessels. The facial nerve may require mobilization from its bony course with anterior displacement. Surgical approaches and their classifications have been extensively described by Fisch. Radiotherapy has also been successfully employed in the management of these tumors [4] (Fig. 12.23).

References

1. Gjuric M, Bilic M (2009) Transmastoid-infralabyrinthine tailored surgery of jugular paragangliomas. Skull Base 19(1):75–83
2. Huang CF, Kondziolka D, Flickinger JC, Lunsford LD (1999) Stereotactic radiosurgery for trigeminal schwannomas. Neurosurgery 45(1):11
3. Lee JD, Kim SH, Song MH, Lee HK, Lee WS (2007) Management of facial nerve schwannoma in patients with favorable facial function. Laryngoscope 117(6): 1063–1068
4. Mazzoni A (2009) The petro-occipital trans-sigmoid approach for lesion of jugular foramen. Skull Base 19(1): 48–57
5. Miller JP, Acar F, Burchiel KJ (2008) Trigeminal neuralgia and vascular compression in patients with trigeminal schwannomas:case report. Neurosurgery 62(4):E974–E975
6. Moiyadi AV, Satish S, Rao G, Santosh V (2008) Multicompartmental trigeminal schwannoma-a clinical report. J Craniofac Surg 19(4):1177–1180
7. Vogal TJ, Bisdas S (2009) Differential diagnosis of jugular foramen lesions. Skull Base 19(1):3–17

Ototoxicity

Core Messages

> › Ototoxicity (both cochlear and vestibular) can occur from systemic and/or topical administration of medications.
>
> › Major ototoxic agents include the aminoglycosides, chemotherapeutic agents (cisplatin) and surgical disinfectants/antiseptics (chlorhexidine, alcohol).
>
> › Individuals with gene defects involving mitochondrial 12S rRNA are exquisitely prone to aminoglycoside ototoxicity.
>
> › Risk factors for systemic aminoglycoside toxicity include a prolonged treatment course (>14 days), elevated serum trough levels, development of renal failure during treatment, concomitant use of other ototoxic medications and a prior history of ototoxicity.

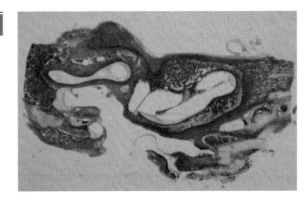

Fig. 13.1 Normal basal turn

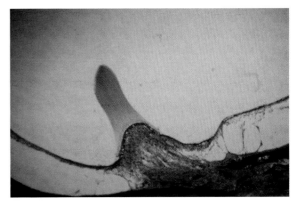

Fig. 13.2 Normal cupula

Ototoxicity can be broadly defined as the tendency of certain substances, either systemic or topical, to cause functional impairment and cellular damage to the tissues of the inner ear and especially to the end organs of the cochlear and vestibular divisions of the eighth cranial nerve. When the cochlea is involved, one primarily identifies a permanent threshold shift in hearing due to the loss of the outer hair cell function. The hearing loss usually begins at the higher frequencies and gradually spreads to involve the lower frequencies. In other words, it progresses from the basal turn of the cochlea toward its apex (Figs.13.1 and 13.2) [1–6].

Major pharmacological groups recognized as being ototoxic to humans include the aminoglycosides, macrolides, cytotoxic agents used in chemotherapy (i.e., cisplatin), loop diuretics, ASA and nonsteroidal anti-inflamatories,

topical antiseptics (i.e., chlorhexidine), quinines, iron chelating agents (i.e., deferoxamine), etc [6].

Major risk factors for aminoglycoside-induced ototoxicity include a prolonged treatment course >14 days, the development of renal failure during treatment, elevated serum aminoglycoside levels (especially preadminstration or trough levels), concomitant use of other ototoxic agents (i.e., diuretics, erythromycin, etc.), and a previous history of ototoxicity. It is

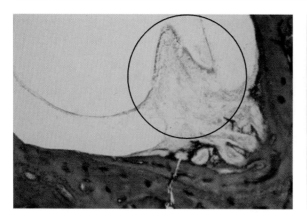

Fig. 13.3 Gentamicin-induced ototoxicity of the ampula. Note the ghost-like image of the crista arising from the loss of type I and type II hair cells. The cupula as well appears to have dissolved. See *circle*

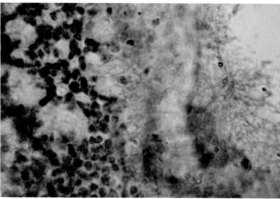

Fig. 13.5 Gentamicin-induced ototoxicity. Hair cell death leads to a vacuolated appearance

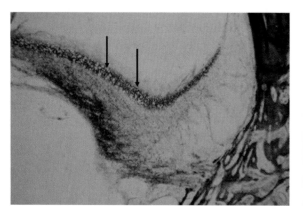

Fig. 13.4 Gentamicin-induced ototoxicity of the utricle. Note the vacuolated appearance of the neuroepithelium. See *arrows*

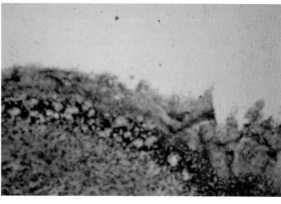

Fig. 13.6 Gentamicin-induced ototoxicity of the crista of the superior semicircular canal. Note the vacuolated appearance of the neuroepithelium

obvious that potentially ototoxic drugs should be carefully monitored especially when used in the presence of any of the risk factors mentioned above. Research in addition has revealed a genetic basis to ototoxicity. Mutations in mitochonrial 12S rRNA appear to especially predispose an individual to ototoxicity from aminoglycosides (Figs. 13.3–13.7) [6, 7].

In addition to the systemic use of potentially ototoxic agents, the topical use of many commercially available otic drop preparations can lead to hearing and vestibular loss. Topical aminoglycosides must be used with care especially if used in long term.

In general, there are several ways through which these topical drugs can reach the inner ear. Portals of entry include the round window membrane (RWM), the annular ligament of the stapes, congenital or acquired microfractures, dehiscences in the otic capsule, and

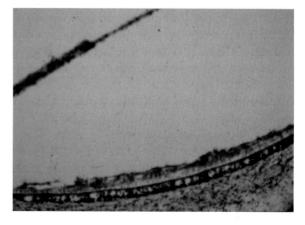

Fig. 13.7 Gentamicin-induced ototoxicity of the saccule

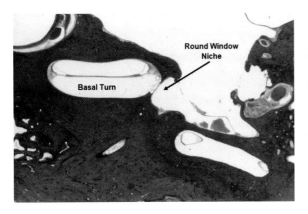

Fig 13.8 Normal appearance of the round window niche and basal turn of cochlea. See *arrow*

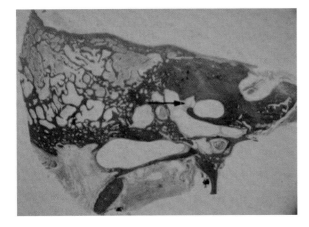

Fig. 13.9 Round window filled with fibrous tissue (see *arrow*)

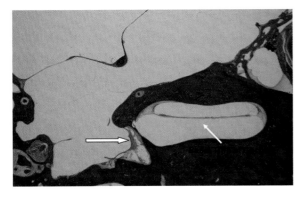

Fig. 13.10 Mucosal web in round window. See *arrow*. Would prevent absorption of ototoxic agents through the RWM

possibly from the systemic uptake of these drugs via the middle ear mucosa.

However, a few anatomical factors and mechanisms exist that serve to prevent absorption into the inner ear (Figs. 13.8–13.10). Those specifically involving the RWM include the fact that:

1. The round window is positioned within a deep niche.
2. In more than 50% of cases, the round window is completely covered by a mucosal fold.
3. Its relative thickness of 65–70 μm is greater compared to the thickness of the RWM in other mammalian species.
4. The presence of mucosal inflammation, debris, and edema that acts as a temporary protective barrier [1, 5].

Since the inner ear contains balance-related (vestibular) and hearing-related (cochlear) end organs, ototoxic drugs not infrequently affect the function of both. When possible, monitoring of the function should be performed. The following tests can be reasonably utilized to evaluate the cochleotoxic effects of the agents with an ototoxic potential. These include:

1. A basic audiologic assessment
2. High-frequency audiometry
3. Oto-acoustic emissions

Bedsides, clinical tests for vestibular function that can be reasonably performed during drug administration include the head shake test, the Halmagyi (high frequency head thrust) maneuver, and the oscillopsia test (which addresses changes in the dynamic visual acuity during active head movement). Formal laboratory tests like electronystamography, rotation chair testing, and posturography can also provide some quantitative information regarding vestibular function.

In general, audiometry should be performed as a base line after 1–2 weeks and after 6 months, especially when a patient is receiving a known ototoxic agent that might affect hearing (i.e., cisplatin)

In an approach to minimize the topical drop ototoxicity, one should clinically consider the following:

1. The use of wicks when treating otitis externa in the presence of a tympanic membrane perforation or defect.
2. Use of drops for as short a duration as necessary (a typical course should last for no longer than 7 days or stop as soon as the otorrhea ceases).
3. Frequent monitoring of the patient's hearing and vestibular function.
4. The choice of topical medications that are unlikely to cause ototoxicity (i.e., floroquinolones) whenever possible (Figs. 13.11–13.13).

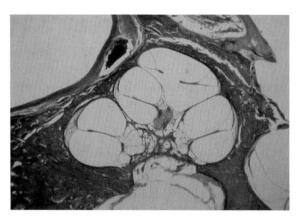

Fig. 13.11 Kanamicin-induced ototoxicity involving the cochlea

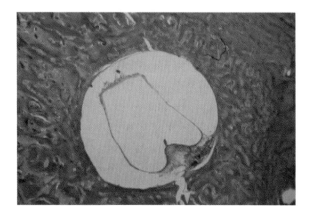

Fig. 13.12 Streptomicin-induced ototoxicity involving the posterior semicircular canal ampulla

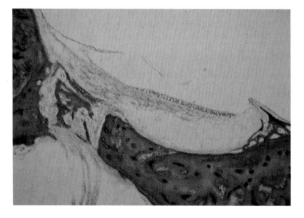

Fig. 13.13 Gentamicin-induced ototoxicity of the saccule

References

1. Andrew P, Walsh, Rory M, Bance, Manohar L, Rutka, John A (1999) Ototoxicity of topical gentamicin preparations. Laryngoscope 109(1):1088–1093
2. Dobie RA, Black FO, Pezsnecker SC, Stallings VL. (2006) Hearing loss in patients with vestibulotoxic reactions to gentamicin therapy. Arch Otolaryngol Head Neck Surg 132(3): 253–257
3. Iwanaga T, Tanaka F, Tsukasaki N, Terakado M, Kaieda S, Takasaki K, Kumagami H, Takahashi H (2006) Does topical application of 5-fluorouracil ointment influence inner ear function? Otolaryngol Head Neck Surg 134(6):961–965
4. Mc Ghan, Lee J, Merchant, Saumil N. (2003) Erythromycin ototoxicity. Otol Neurotol 24(4):701–702
5. Pappas S, Nikolopoulos TP, Korres S, Papacharalampous G, Tzangarulakis A, Ferekidis E (2006) Topical antibiotic ear drops: are they safe? Int J Clin Pract 60(9):1115–1119
6. Roland PS, John A, Rutka, MD (2004) Ototoxicity. BC Decker, ON
7. Rodriguez-Ballesteros M, Oltare M, Aguirre L A, Galan F, Galan R, Vallejo L A, Navas C, Villamar M, Moreno-Pelayo, Moreno F, del Castillo I. (2006) Molecular and clinical inherited non-syndromic hearing loss caused by the 1494c- > T mutation in the mitochondrial 12S rRNA gene. J Med Genet 43(11):e54

Index

Printing and Binding: Stürtz GmbH, Würzburg